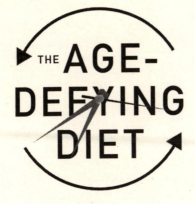

THE AGE-
DEFYING
DIET

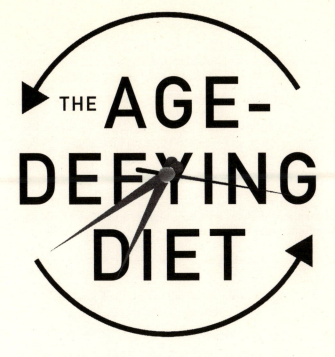

THE AGE-DEFYING DIET

OUTSMART YOUR METABOLISM TO LOSE WEIGHT—UP TO 20 POUNDS IN 21 DAYS!—AND TURN BACK THE CLOCK

CAROLINE APOVIAN, MD

This edition first published in Great Britain in 2015 by
Orion
an imprint of the Orion Publishing Group Ltd
Carmelite House, 50 Victoria Embankment,
London EC4Y 0DZ
An Hachette UK Company

1 3 5 7 9 10 8 6 4 2

A CIP catalogue record for this book is available
from the British Library.

Trade Paperback ISBN: 9781409158257

Printed in Great Britain by CPI Group (UK) Ltd, Croydon, CR0 4YY

The Orion Publishing Group's policy is to use papers that are natural,
renewable and recyclable and made from wood grown in sustainable forests.
The logging and manufacturing processes are expected to conform to the
environmental regulations of the country of origin.

*Every effort has been made to ensure that the information in this book
is accurate. The information will be relevant to the majority of people
but may not be applicable in each individual case, so it is advised that
professional medical advice is obtained for specific health matters. Neither
the publisher nor author accept any legal responsibility for any personal
injury or other damage or loss arising from the use or misuse of the
information in this book. Anyone making a change in their diet should
consult their GP, especially if pregnant, infirm, elderly or under 16.*

Every effort has been made to fulfil requirements with regard
to reproducing copyright material. The author and publisher will
be glad to rectify any omissions at the earliest opportunity.

To my John and my Philip—
may you stay forever young

Acknowledgments

This book could not have been written without the help and dedication of a team of fabulous people around me sharing their expertise and enthusiasm. Thank you to Frances Sharpe and Harriet Bell for their ability to put it all together, and to Trevor Wisdom and Rochelle Schmidt for developing such creative and delicious recipes.

Thank you to Wayne Westcott, whose knowledge of the science of physical fitness is unsurpassed, and Rita La Rosa Loud, who makes it all happen in the fitness world.

A big thank you to the whole team at Grand Central Publishing, especially Sarah Pelz, Matthew Ballast, and Diana Baroni, who are always ready to offer a solution for every little thing. Thank you as well to Sarah Christensen Fu and Ellen Schwartz.

Thank you to my Boston University School of Medicine team, Mitali Shah, RD, and Ashley Bourland, who checked every recipe to make sure they were right and missed nothing.

Thank you to David Blackburn and Rod Egger, who brought the Science-Smart SuperCharged Smoothie Mix line to a new level with the Age-Defying Diet program. Thank you to George Blackburn, my mentor and dear friend, who always steered me in the right direction, and sees above everyone else.

And a special thank you to Philip Lief, the other person who also sees above everyone else!

Thank you to my father, Dr. John Apovian, for believing in me (always), and to my mother, Ines Chinni Apovian, the real creator of the Age-Defying Diet. And last but not least, thank you to my little family, the Baker boys, Gus, John, and Philip, for supporting me no matter what.

Contents

Introduction

When I saw my patient Leslie walking through my office recently, I thought she'd just come by to gush about her continuing weight loss. I always encourage patients to stay in touch, and love to see their progress and successes.

When Leslie first came to me as a patient, she was a 47-year-old sales executive and mother of two who wanted to lose the 35 pounds she had gained over the past years. I introduced her to my Age-Defying Diet program, a powerful, three-week program designed to re-ignite your metabolism and fight aging. Two months later, she had lost 28 pounds and trimmed 4½ inches off her waist. The program clearly worked for Leslie. Now in my office, six months after she reached her goal weight, she looked terrific in her slim-fitting jeans.

"So, what brings you in today?" I asked her.

"Oh, I'm not here for me." She laughed. "I'm here with him."

As if on cue, a man strolled into my office. Leslie introduced her husband, Jeff. Jeff was 48 years old and complained of low energy and little, if any, interest in having sex with his wife. He often felt down in the dumps, especially after he started taking prescription medicine for high blood pressure and high cholesterol.

"Look," Jeff said. "Leslie seems like she's in her prime; she's healthier and happier than ever. I'm the old guy at home on the couch and she's out playing touch football in the yard with the kids every weekend. I'm ready to lose this gut and start enjoying our personal and family time together again."

When Leslie first came to see me, she was very worried about signs of perimenopause. She told me about her hot flashes, how she was having trouble remembering everyday things—*Why did I walk into this room? Where are my car keys? What's that woman's name in the accounting department?*—and felt like she had a serious case of "brain fog." But these things weren't what was really bothering her. It was her weight, she said, that was making her look and feel out of sorts.

Leslie was no stranger to trying to lose weight. Like many women, she'd been doing it for most of her life, and she was good at it. Whenever she put on an extra 15 or 20 pounds, she used a few tried-and-true dieting tactics—eating fewer calories and ramping up her cardio workouts—until she was able to fit back into her skinny jeans. Her low-calorie, high-cardio strategy always worked in the past. Leslie slimmed down for her wedding at age 27 by spending hours on the treadmill. Skipping dessert and wine helped her get back into shape for her 20th high school reunion in her late 30s, and helped her fit into a sleek, fitted little black dress she wore for her 15th wedding anniversary when she was 42. But now her body was not responding the same way. She felt overweight, unattractive, and unsexy. Her once active sex drive had disappeared.

When I first met Leslie, she was frustrated.

"This doesn't make any sense," she told me during our first meeting. "I've never had a problem losing weight. I've been doing the same thing I've always done when I need to lose a few pounds. But it isn't working anymore."

All too often, I hear this from people who come to my office at Boston University Medical Center, where I'm director of the Nutrition and Weight Management Center.

I explained to Leslie that her former diet strategy, a low-calorie diet, actually lowered her metabolism. This occurs because your body tries to maintain a certain body weight set point—the number you weigh give or take a few pounds. When you eat fewer calories, your body counteracts the lower energy intake by decreasing its resting metabolic rate. On top of that, her low-calorie diet robbed Leslie's body of lean muscle tissue because she was eating less protein, which caused a further drop in the effectiveness of her metabolism. Her all-cardio exercise routine burned some fat, but it also burned all-important muscle tissue and caused her metabolism to become even more sluggish. At her first visit, I asked her to keep a food diary so I could see what she was eating every day. Her food diary showed me that she occasionally skipped breakfast and ate pasta for dinner at least three times a week, because it was quick to put together. She had a salad just two or three times a week. As a result of her eating habits, her diet was deficient in several key nutrients—iron, vitamin B$_{12}$, and vitamin C because she didn't eat many fruits and vegetables—all of which contribute to increased muscle loss and a slower metabolism, resulting in extra pounds. During Leslie's physical exam, I noticed that her skin, especially on her hands, feet, and elbows, was exceptionally dry. When I asked her about her dry skin, Leslie said she used an entire large bottle of moisturizer every month. I explained to her that on the Age-Defying Diet, she would be eating foods rich in essential amino acids—proteins, safflower oil, and a variety of green vegetables—that would make her dry skin soft and hydrated again.

I told her that thanks to hormonal changes, your metabolism slows down as you get older. In women, ovaries start producing less estrogen at the onset of menopause, and in men, testosterone levels drop starting at age 30, though men may not feel the difference until their 40s. In women and men, these hormonal changes affect metabolism and lead to excess weight, especially in the midsection. For example, fat cells produce estrogen. When a woman's ovaries start to slow down estrogen production, her fat cells try to pick up the slack, especially the fat cells in the abdominal area. The bigger those fat cells become, the more estrogen they can make, so the body conspires to plump up those fat cells.

In men, it's a vicious cycle. Lower amounts of testosterone are produced, which drains energy and often leads to weight gain. Excess fat compounds the problem by decreasing testosterone levels even further. My male patients don't like it when I explain that belly fat actually converts testosterone to estrogen, contributing to an overall "softer" appearance.

I talked with Jeff about his eating and exercising habits. It didn't take long to realize that Jeff was going through the same metabolic slump that Leslie had experienced. He was confused and frustrated—why was his body all of a sudden rebelling? He told me he was eating the same things and the same amount of food he'd always consumed but was suddenly gaining weight. What was different now?

The answers aren't simple, but it all has to do with your age and your metabolism. In a cruel twist of biology, your metabolism begins to slow down once you reach 30. That's partly because muscle loss, called sarcopenia in medical-speak, comes naturally with aging. It is the primary reason for metabolic slowdown and why it becomes harder to lose weight with each passing year. Starting around age 30, you lose about 1 percent of your muscle mass each year, and when you reach your mid-40s this process speeds up. Muscle burns more calories than fat, so the greater your muscle mass, the higher your metabolism; muscle loss plays a direct role in your body's fat-burning abilities.

The other problem is that the lost lean muscle tissue is replaced by fat. Losing just 5 pounds of muscle means that 5 pounds of flab will replace it—usually right around the waistline. A little 5-pound addition doesn't sound dramatic, but combine it with hormonal changes, and you're right on track for metabolism meltdown.

In Jeff's case, by eating "the same things" he always had, he wasn't consuming enough of the specific nutrients necessary to reverse the muscle loss process, which leads to a slower metabolism and more stored fat. Second, because his metabolism had lowered, he was burning fewer calories than he used to. When he continued to eat the same quantities of food, more pounds just piled on.

It felt great to give Jeff the good news—the same good news I'd given Leslie a few months back. I walked him through my Age-Defying Diet program, explaining that the plan is designed to help people boost and reset their metabolism.

"Follow the plan and you will lose weight and feel vast improvements to your health," I assured him. "It worked for Leslie, and it can work for you, Jeff."

It's easy to understand how frustrating a slow metabolism can be, but it doesn't mean that you just have to accept weight gain, or that there's nothing you can do to reverse the metabolic aging process. Your metabolism might be low now, but that doesn't mean it has to be stuck there forever. You can reverse the process, boost your vitality, and earn a younger metabolic age with the Age-Defying Diet. It has already helped thousands of people just like Leslie and Jeff take years off their metabolic age and subsequently boost energy, improve memory, enhance moods, bring the spark back to their sex lives, shed fat, and lose up to 20 pounds in three weeks!

Three Weeks to a Younger, Slimmer You

As one of the world's leading researchers on obesity and weight loss, I'm privy to—and sometimes directly involved in—the most cutting-edge research on the science of losing weight. If you're in your 30s, 40s, 50s, and beyond—and, like Leslie and Jeff, struggling with the weight gain and hormonal changes that come with aging—then this book is designed for you. Based on the latest findings and my own clinical experience with thousands of people who have successfully lost weight, I have created a three-step program for losing weight, turning back the clock, and lowering your metabolic age:

• **Reboot** lasts just seven days and focuses on drinking Super-Charged Smoothies in addition to high-protein meals to lose fat. You'll do strength-training exercises for nine minutes two times during the week to build muscle.

• **Recharge** lasts two weeks and keeps your metabolism in high gear by offering a diet of protein- and nutrient-rich whole foods, Super-Charged Smoothies, and SuperCharged Soups. You will be doing strength training exercises for only 18 minutes two times per week.

• **Revitalize** is your solution to feeling younger and staying slimmer for life. It will keep your metabolic age younger than your chronological age and keep those pounds from building back up with great meal plans and by exercising for only 30 minutes twice a week.

These simple steps will re-ignite your sluggish and stubborn metabolism.

I developed the Age-Defying Diet primarily to help people with slow metabolisms reverse the process in order to lose unhealthy fat. But rapid weight loss, increased energy, and a younger metabolic age aren't the only benefits that come with this program. Just ask Leslie and Jeff.

Leslie told me she now experiences fewer hot flashes, and has no problem remembering where she left her keys. Her skin is soft and healthy-looking, and she no longer feels like she's suffering from "brain fog." Even better, her friends tell her she looks years younger. "They even asked me if I'd had any cosmetic procedures done," she said, beaming.

Jeff, who started the program the very next day, lost 20 pounds in 21 days. He went from a 38-inch to a 34-inch waist and says he has more energy than ever. His blue moods have lessened, and he received great news after his last health checkup. "My blood pressure was normal, and my cholesterol was back in the healthy range, so I was able to stop taking my medications," he added. "That's a relief. Nothing makes me feel older than having an entire pharmacy in my medicine cabinet. We no longer have to plan ahead when we want to have sex. Those little blue pills are a thing of the past."

How to Use This Book

In chapter 1: Metabolism Meltdown, I explain in easy-to-understand terms what causes your metabolism to slow down. You'll discover how this medically sound three-week program is designed to reboot your metabolism and turn back the clock on your metabolic age.

Chapter 2: Eating to Boost Your Metabolism introduces the foods that will re-ignite your stalled metabolism so you can start burning fat, resculpting your body, and enjoying the many other benefits of a younger metabolic age. You'll discover why you need to eat more protein than you think to fuel your metabolism and how to make intermittent fasting even more effective at sparking your metabolism. Intermittent fasting refers to alternating periods of eating and not eating solid foods, or fasting. Cravings and hunger are the reason that most people fail when it comes to traditional low-calorie diets. With the Age-Defying Diet, my protein-rich smoothies keep you full and satisfied until it's time for the next meal.

While women and men are physiologically alike in many ways, they do have significant hormonal differences that are detailed in chapter 3: Women and Men: Individual Metabolic Needs. Foods that women and men should and shouldn't eat are listed.

Chapter 4: The Age-Defying Diet is the heart of the program. I explain what to drink—SuperCharged Smoothies and Super-Charged Soups—and the rich whole-food meals you'll eat to lose weight quickly and effectively.

Chapter 5: The Age-Defying Workout explains the simple, short, strength-training exercises you'll be doing to build lean muscle and burn fat. Even if you've never exercised before, step-by-step instructions and photographs accompany each exercise.

Learn why getting a good night's sleep is absolutely essential to rebooting and maintaining a revved-up metabolism in chapter 6: How Sleep Affects Your Metabolism and Your Weight. I include tips like keeping your room as dark as possible, drinking sleep-inducing smoothies, and other suggestions to help you get the shut-eye you need to enhance metabolic repair without the use of pharmaceutical sleep aids.

Chapter 7: The Age-Defying Diet Day by Day offers a meal-by-meal blueprint with suggested SuperCharged Smoothies, Super-Charged Soups, and whole-food meals.

In chapters 8, 9, and 10, you'll find recipes for those Super-Charged Smoothies, SuperCharged Soups, satisfying whole-food meals, and desserts. Delicious and filling, they all contain the right amounts of protein, calories, and other nutrients for fast, healthy weight loss.

That's everything you need to reboot your metabolism. Just give me three weeks to show you how to lower your metabolic age, so you look and feel years younger and lose weight fast.

How to Calculate Your Metabolic Age

Take this simple quiz and see what age your metabolism is functioning at now. Just add (or subtract) the number next to your answers to (or from) your chronological age. Don't be discouraged by the results. I guarantee that after just three weeks on the Age-Defying Diet, you will see a major improvement in your metabolic age, your waistline, your energy, and your health.

1. Determine your BMI (Body Mass Index). Find your BMI on the chart on pages 298–9.
   - If your BMI is: 18 to 22, subtract 2.
   - If your BMI is: 22 to 25, subtract 1.
   - If your BMI is: 25 to 27, add 0.
   - If your BMI is: 27 to 30, add 2.
   - If your BMI is: 30 to 35, add 4.
   - If your BMI is: 35 to 40, add 6.
   - If your BMI is: over 40, add 8.
2. What shape is your body?
   - If you're shaped like an apple or a rectangle, add 2.
   - If you're shaped like a pear or an hourglass, subtract 1.
3. Do you have Type 2 diabetes?
   - If yes (fasting blood glucose greater than 100) or if you take medication for Type 2 diabetes, add 2.

4. Do you have high blood pressure?
    - If yes (blood pressure greater than or equal to 140/90), the doctor told you that you need medication, and/or you are on medication, add 3.
5. Do you have high blood lipids or cholesterol?
    - If yes (LDL cholesterol greater than or equal to 160 or HDL less than 35) or you take medication, add 3.
6. Do you smoke tobacco?
    - If the answer is yes, add 8.
7. How many alcoholic beverages do you drink every day?
    - If you're a woman who drinks more than 1 drink a day, add 4.
    - If you're a man who drinks more than 2 drinks a day, add 4.
8. How many servings of fruits and vegetables do you eat every day?
    - If you eat fewer than 2 servings of fruits and vegetables per day, add 2.
    - If you eat 2 to 4 servings of fruits and vegetables per day, add 1.
    - If you eat 4 to 6 servings of fruits and vegetables per day, subtract 1.
    - If you eat 6 to 8 servings of fruits and vegetables per day, subtract 2.
    - If you eat more than 8 servings of fruits and vegetables per day, subtract 3.
9. How often do you exercise?
    - If you never exercise, add 2.
    - If you exercise 1 to 2 times per week, subtract 1.
    - If you exercise 3 to 4 times per week, subtract 2.
    - If you exercise 5 to 7 times per week, subtract 4.
10. How much water or other liquids that contain no calories do you drink per day?
    - If you are a woman and you drink 7 or more glasses of water or other liquids that have no calories per day, subtract 2.

- If you are a woman and you drink more than 5 but fewer than 7 glasses of water or other liquids that have no calories per day, add 2.
- If you are a woman and you drink fewer than 5 glasses of water or other liquids that have no calories per day, add 4.
- If you are a woman and drink mainly juice or sugar-sweetened sodas or beverages, add 4.
- If you are a man and you drink 12 or more glasses of water or other liquids that have no calories per day, subtract 2.
- If you are a man and you drink more than 8 but fewer than 12 glasses of water or other liquids that have no calories per day, add 2.
- If you are a man and you drink fewer than 8 glasses of water or other liquids that have no calories per day, add 4.
- If you are a man and drink mainly juice or sugar-sweetened sodas or beverages, add 4.

11. How much protein do you eat?
    - If you eat protein or a complete protein substitute at every meal or most meals daily, subtract 4.
    - If you eat protein at one meal daily, subtract 2.
    - If you eat protein twice per week, add 0.
    - If you eat protein once per week, add 2.

12. What do you think your daily stress level is?
    - High stress, add 2.
    - Moderate stress, add 1.
    - Mild stress, add 0.
    - No stress, subtract 1.

13. How many hours of uninterrupted sleep do you average every night?
    - Fewer than 5 hours, add 2.
    - 5 to 6 hours, add 1.
    - 6 to 7 hours, subtract 1.
    - 7 to 9 hours, subtract 2.
    - More than 9 hours, add 2.

Your chronological age is_____

Plus or minus the number from above_____

Your metabolic age is_____

I will show you how to outsmart your metabolism so you can turn back the clock and lose weight in just three weeks.

Retake this quiz after three weeks on the Age-Defying Diet and you will see how successful you've been!

Your metabolic age after three weeks on the Age-Defying Diet:

CHAPTER 1

_____

Metabolism Meltdown

It's no secret that your body undergoes significant changes as you age. You discover that you can't eat or drink whatever you want or as much as you want without gaining weight, especially extra fat around your middle. You find that those no-fail diet tricks you used to pull no longer work, and your usual workout routine—running on a treadmill or using an elliptical trainer—is not as effective as it was when you were younger. And your energy levels? Well, they definitely aren't what they used to be. By nine o'clock, you're completely exhausted, yet once you climb into bed it takes hours until you fall into a deep sleep. If you're a woman, symptoms of perimenopause or menopause, such as hot flashes and night sweats, make it even more difficult to get a good night's sleep—if you get any at all. If you're a man, you notice that your sex drive isn't what it once was. All of these things add up and suddenly, before you know it, the weight has crept up on you.

What's going on here?

As you get older, your metabolism slows down, and as a result your body and brain don't perform as they once did. While a metabolic slowdown eventually happens to everyone as the years go by, don't give up now. There is a way to rejuvenate your metabolism, feel and look younger, and be thinner.

Based on my successful work with thousands of men and women as director of the Nutrition and Weight Management Center, Boston

University Medical Center, the Age-Defying Diet shows how you can once again have a metabolism that lets you burn fat, lose weight, maintain brain function, feel energetic, and keep your immune system strong.

The Metabolic Aging Game

Metabolism is a complex bodily process that uses hormones and enzymes to convert food into fuel. The rate—fast or slow—at which your body burns that fuel is essential to every function your body performs.

As you get older, your metabolism ages, too. In fact, your metabolism actually ages faster than the number of candles on your birthday cake—slowing down by 5 percent each decade. By age 45, you're burning about 200 fewer calories per day than you did when you were 25. While that may not sound like much, it could mean a weight gain of as much as 12 pounds each year. Most likely, the extra weight will settle in right around your waistline and belly. For some people, the healthy eating and exercise habits they have been following for years no longer work no matter how hard they try. Whether it's trying every new fad diet that comes along, eating fewer carbs, counting calories, or exercising for hours, they still gain weight. Others have a metabolism that has always functioned at a slower pace, which explains why they've struggled with weight problems for their entire adult lives.

To understand how your metabolism can be outsmarted to help you lose weight, you need to become familiar with the powerful forces at work inside your body. First, you need to understand what's keeping your metabolism from operating at its best. Then I will show you how to regain control over your metabolic age and your weight, so you can feel fantastic.

How Does the Age-Defying Diet Work?

Following the Age-Defying Diet is like hitting a REBOOT button in your body by making specific changes to what you eat and how you exercise. As you age, you lose muscle mass. The only way to reverse muscle loss is increase your muscle mass by reversing your metabolic age. Almost from the minute you drink your first age-defying Super-Charged Smoothie or finish your first bowl of SuperCharged Soup, you'll notice that you feel and look better every day. After three weeks on the program, you will lose up to 20 pounds of fat, especially around the midsection of your body. In a matter of days, your clothes will be noticeably looser and your energy levels will soar.

The Muscle Loss–Metabolic Aging Connection

I tell my patients that if they don't start eating a proper diet and exercising appropriately by the age of 30, their muscle tissue will begin to shrink by about 1 percent each year. By the time they reach their mid-40s, muscle begins to erode at an accelerated pace. By age 70, men and women can lose as much as 2 percent of muscle tissue per year for a total loss of 30 percent! Significant muscle loss can lead to poor balance, falls, and fractures.

When lean muscle tissue is lost, it is typically replaced by fat on your middle or on your hips and thighs. When 40-year-old Marlene came to see me, she weighed 145 pounds, the same as she did in her 20s. While her weight was the same, she wondered how it was possible that she had added 4 inches to her waistline through the years. I explained to her that when she was in her 20s, she might have had a 26 percent body fat percentage, which means 105 pounds were lean body mass, muscles, bones, organs, and other tissues. Now that Marlene was 40 and her weight was steady at 145 pounds, measurements showed us that her body fat percentage had climbed to 32 percent. She was now carrying around about 46 pounds of fat and just 99 pounds of lean body mass. That was a 12-pound increase in her flab-to-muscle ratio!

The transition from lean tissue to more body fat doesn't show up on a scale that only measures pounds. After all, 6 pounds of fat and 6 pounds of muscle each weighs 6 pounds, but they have different amounts of mass and can *dramatically* change the shape of your body and your well-being. That additional fat on you slows down your metabolism and makes you feel hungry, weak, tired, sluggish, and, let's face it, *fat*.

Although your belly is the primary target for the increase in fat that comes with a loss of lean muscle, it isn't the only one. Some fat actually infiltrates your decreasing muscle tissue. (Even though some fat cells can insinuate themselves near muscle cells, a fat cell is always a fat cell and a muscle cell is always a muscle cell. One can't change into the other.) Imaging studies reveal that the more fat you have on your body, the more fat you have in your muscles, too. This depletes your muscles' calorie-burning capacity and further slows down your metabolism.

The decrease in the quality of your muscle fibers also leaves you feeling weaker, which usually makes you less inclined to engage in physical activity. This helps explain why older adults tend to be less active. Among all U.S. adults over the age of 18, nearly 80 percent aren't getting enough physical activity, and more than 70 percent aren't meeting the minimum muscle-training requirements, according to the Centers for Disease Control and Prevention. These statistics get worse the older you get. While most people aren't getting *enough* exercise, nearly 30 percent of middle-aged men and women aren't getting *any* exercise, meaning they engage in no physical activity whatsoever. Talk about a recipe for metabolic disaster!

The hormonal changes that come with the passage of time in both women and men cause a biological chain reaction that compounds the problem and can make it seem impossible to shed extra weight or feel and look as you once did. While women and men share many metabolic issues, they have different health and hormonal concerns when rebooting their metabolisms and losing weight.

MUSCLE LOSS–METABOLIC AGING CYCLE

Here's a diagram showing the endless cycle of a slowing metabolism:

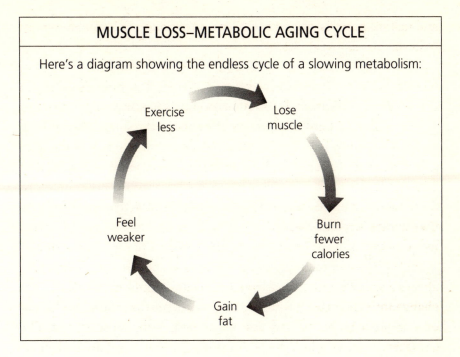

REVERSING THE CYCLE WITH THE AGE-DEFYING DIET PLAN

With the Age-Defying Diet program, I'll show how you can reverse the harmful cycle above in just three weeks:

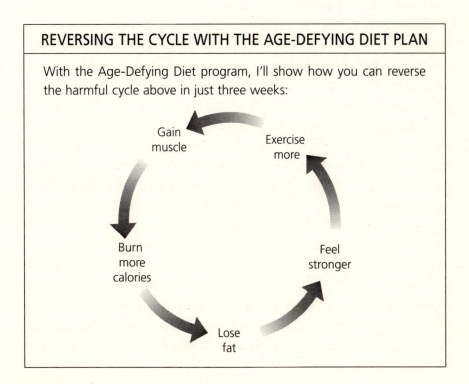

See chapter 3: Women and Men: Individual Metabolic Needs (page 41).

Health Conditions That Cause Metabolism Meltdown

Aging, hormonal changes, and muscle loss also contribute to metabolism meltdown via insulin resistance and chronic inflammation. Many of my patients are surprised to learn how these conditions sabotage their metabolism.

Insulin Resistance

Insulin is a hormone produced by the pancreas. It helps your body use glucose for energy and also helps your body store excess glucose in fat cells. In a healthy body, when you eat starches, your body converts them to glucose, which raises your blood sugar levels. In response, your pancreas releases insulin to escort that glucose out of the bloodstream and into the muscles, liver, or fat cells. With insulin resistance, your body produces insulin but doesn't use the hormone efficiently, so your body keeps producing insulin. High levels of insulin can cause water retention and make you feel and look bloated. Insulin resistance is also linked to being overweight and having extra belly fat. The more insulin-resistant you are, the more weight you will gain, and the more likely it is that you will develop Type 2 diabetes. The first thing any doctor will tell a pre-diabetic or diabetic patient to do is to lose weight. The Age-Defying Diet lets you accomplish that, so your body uses its insulin more effectively.

Chronic Inflammation

If you cut yourself while chopping an onion, your body automatically increases blood flow to the injured area. You know your immune system is hard at work, fighting infection when the cut area turns red. That's called acute inflammation, and it's essential to the body's healing process. On the other hand, chronic, or systemic, inflammation occurs when the body's immune system tries to fight an infection that isn't there. No one is certain what causes chronic inflammation, but it is at the heart of conditions like rheumatoid arthritis, gastrointestinal illnesses such as Crohn's disease and colitis, cancer, and insulin resistance. Insulin resistance can fuel systemic inflammation, making it even harder for you to lose weight. I have written more than 100 articles on weight loss, muscle metabolism, and the relationship between insulin resistance and inflammation that have been published in leading medical journals. My research has consistently found that in people with insulin resistance, the body's immune system cells pump out substances called cytokines that promote inflammation. As mentioned above, the best way to fight insulin resistance is to maintain a lean body. I am currently involved in exciting research that is looking to find an OFF switch to stop the release of these harmful cytokines, which may reduce inflammation, insulin resistance, and obesity.

Losing fat and building muscle with the Age-Defying Diet can help in the battle against debilitating chronic inflammation.

Gut Health

As you age, your microbiome, which is all of the microflora—good and bad bacteria—that work together in your body, changes as well. When the production of gut hormones decreases, you may become constipated or develop acid reflux. Gut microbiomes are also different in those who are obese versus lean, perhaps due to a diet high in fat and processed carbohydrates and low in lean protein. No matter what the causes, the Age-Defying Diet will help keep your gut hormones in balance.

Brain Function

Have you ever had a "senior moment," when you forgot the name of the restaurant where you ate last night, or where you left your eyeglasses? You aren't alone, and you aren't imagining it. Brain function is closely tied to your metabolic age.

Age-related changes occurring in the brain can also result in emotional upheaval, leaving you feeling irritated, angry, or depressed. Often these mood issues are related to your fluctuating hormones, especially cortisol, which is called the stress hormone. As your levels rise and fall, hormone receptors in the brain take note of the changes and alter the production of neurochemicals involved in mood stability. This plays a role in those mood swings.

If you're more forgetful, more easily distracted, or more emotional, these states can lead to lifestyle choices that cause your metabolism to age more rapidly. Instead of eating lean proteins, fruits, and vegetables to stoke your metabolism, you head to the nearest drive-through fast-food joint. Or you stress-eat, stuffing yourself with your favorite foods. Even worse, you find yourself skipping breakfast and lunch, and then sit down to a huge meal with a few glasses of wine at the end of the day. Rather than heading to the gym for your regular workout, because you're wiped out from work and other responsibilities, you plant yourself in front of the TV or curl up with your favorite mobile device for hours at night. All of these lifestyle choices can impair a healthy, properly functioning metabolism. The Age-Defying Diet tackles these problems with a program that boosts your metabolism and cuts years off your metabolic age.

Six Simple Steps to Revitalize Your Metabolism

Now that you understand why your metabolism is sluggish and causing you to gain weight, here are the six things you need to do to rejuvenate your body and your brain:

1. Eat More Protein, Vegetables, and Fruits

Not eating enough protein, cutting out all carbohydrates as some diets suggest, or otherwise shunning specific foods or food groups to lose weight can backfire on your metabolism. For example, a lack of health-promoting carbohydrates—such as vegetables, fruits, and small amounts of whole grains—is associated with an increased risk for inflammation and insulin resistance, and, as a result, will slow down your metabolism and cause you to gain weight.

2. Eat Your Essential Amino Acids

Amino acids are the building blocks of protein, and they're responsible for generating, regenerating, and repairing all the cells and tissues in your body, muscles, and brain. The best sources for amino acids are meat, fish, eggs, and other protein-rich food. The Age-Defying Diet guarantees that you'll eat the right kind of good food to get the necessary amounts of these critical nutrients.

3. Eat to Maintain Hormonal Balance

Some foods can help ward off the symptoms associated with the age-related hormonal changes in both men and women, while others can worsen any hormonal changes already taking place.

4. Eat the Right Foods to Fill You Up

If you're still eating the same amount of food you ate when you were in your 20s, you're eating too much. With the natural decline in muscle mass, dwindling hormone levels, and slowing metabolism, you need fewer calories as you get older, especially if you aren't exercising to counteract these changes. Continuing to eat what you've always eaten is a surefire recipe for gaining that potbelly. The Super-Charged Smoothies, SuperCharged Soups, and whole-food meals in the Age-Defying Diet will keep you satisfied, prevent cravings, and help keep off those extra pounds.

If you've been following a low-calorie eating plan for an extended period of time, or you jump on and off the traditional diet wagon, you may have inadvertently slowed down your metabolism. When your body isn't getting adequate nutrition for energy, it robs tissue from your muscles to use for energy. This hastens the muscle loss process and brings your metabolism into meltdown mode. The Age-Defying Diet offers plenty of delicious, satisfying food. By knowing what to eat and when and having every meal planned out, you won't be hungry and make poor food choices throughout the day.

5. Exercise Properly to Lose Weight

Trying to lose fat by doing hours of cardio can actually put you on the fast track to metabolism slowdown. During aerobic exercise, muscle proteins are broken down for energy. Some cardio activity is good for you, but you should be careful not to overdo it. In chapter 5, you'll learn simple exercises to spark weight loss and build muscle tissue. You'll do exercises for different amounts of time, adding more exercises as you progress through the program. During Reboot, you'll spend just nine minutes twice a week doing two exercises. In Recharge, you'll exercise for 18 minutes twice a week doing four exercises. In Revitalize, you'll maintain your success by spending 30 minutes twice a week doing five exercises. In addition to strength training, keep up or include other activities—walking, swimming, cycling, basketball. The main message here? Keep moving!

6. Get More Quality Sleep

If you're anything like my patients, you're probably trying to do it all up until the very last second of the day. These are the years when you have to balance career and work responsibilities, take care of your children, care for aging parents, and still find time to enjoy your own life. With all of this on your plate, chances are high that stress hormones, such as cortisol, are kicking in and preventing you from getting a good night's sleep. In addition, changing hormonal levels are also affecting your sleep patterns and causing you to drag your feet throughout the day.

Not getting adequate shut-eye disrupts the natural muscle repair and regeneration process. This contributes to even more muscle loss and more fat gain. And did you know that your appetite hormones are primarily regulated while you sleep? Just one night of tossing and turning can turn up your hunger hormones and lead you to consume more calories. A lack of sleep actually alters the biology of your fat cells, according to a study published in the *Annals of Internal Medicine* (2012). When people slept for just four and a half hours for four consecutive nights, their fat cells were 30 percent less sensitive to the fat-burning hormone insulin. As you read earlier in this chapter, this metabolic change is associated with an increased risk for insulin resistance, which is linked to more belly fat. According to one of the study's authors, just four nights of restricted sleep is the equivalent of adding 10 to 20 years to your metabolic age.

The Age-Defying Diet shows that by drinking my Sleepytime Smoothies and eating the right kinds of foods, you'll get a good night's rest. But for those who need additional help getting those much-needed seven to eight hours of sleep, I have some surefire natural remedies in chapter 6 to help you sleep like a baby. Every night.

Reversing Metabolism Meltdown

Now you understand how your body, hormones, and metabolism conspire to prevent you from losing that not-so-delicious muffin top or love handle. Even if you are in full metabolism meltdown mode, it's not too late to reverse the process and lose the weight. You'll see how the Age-Defying Diet will help you boost declining hormones naturally, put a halt to muscle loss, and begin reversing conditions like chronic inflammation and insulin resistance. By making simple lifestyle changes, you can take years off your metabolic age and inches off your middle. Suddenly you'll have that waistline back like you did in your 20s—maybe even better.

CHAPTER 2

Eating to Boost Your Metabolism

What you eat and drink can either hasten the metabolic meltdown process or boost your metabolism to give you a younger metabolic age than your chronological age. In this chapter, you'll discover how making the right food choices can change your biochemistry and help you fight the battle against that bulging midsection. You'll discover how the foods you'll be eating on this plan will help balance your hunger and stress hormones to reverse the situations that promote fat storage and help you lose the weight you hate—all without feeling hungry or deprived. By changing what you eat, your memory and moods will improve and you'll feel more rejuvenated and reinvigorated than you have in years.

The Power of Protein

Consuming an adequate amount of protein is the key to rebooting your metabolism and sparking weight loss. Why is protein so important if you want to turn back the clock on metabolic aging? Protein helps maintain lean muscle tissue, which promotes a cascade of biological benefits.

Protein and Your Muscles

In the 1970s, Dr. George Blackburn began conducting scientific research on the impact of protein consumption on weight loss and muscle preservation. One of his first studies, published in the *Journal of the American Medical Association*, reported that a low-calorie diet that included 1.5 grams of protein per kilogram of *ideal* body weight per day provided safe and effective weight loss. Follow-up studies went even further to isolate the impact of protein consumption on weight loss and the maintenance of muscle tissue. One study in the *Journal of Clinical Investigation* compared the effects of eating 0.8 versus 1.5 grams of protein per kilogram of ideal body weight per day. Consuming the lower amount of protein resulted in biological conditions indicating that muscle loss was occurring. Eating the higher amount of protein indicated optimum conditions for muscle maintenance. The bottom line? Less protein, less muscle tissue, lower metabolism. More protein, more muscle tissue, faster metabolism, less fat.

Researchers continue to build on Dr. Blackburn's science by investigating the effects of protein intake specifically among people who are middle-aged or beyond. I am one of those researchers. I'm currently involved in a study that focuses on the protein requirements of men in midlife. Preliminary results indicate that these men need to eat even more than the currently recommended amount of protein per kilogram of ideal body weight per day in order to maintain lean tissue.

You don't have to reach middle age to start pumping up your protein intake. Did you know that when you try to lose weight with most traditional diet and exercise plans, you tend to lose muscle tissue, rather than fat tissue? In fact, many scientists believe that *significant* muscle loss is inevitable while dieting. This doesn't have to be the case. A 2013 study in the *FASEB Journal* has confirmed that doubling the recommended daily intake (RDI) for protein helps protect lean tissue while promoting fat loss.

Protein: A Smart Way to Enhance Brain Function

You don't need cognitive tests or brain-imaging scans to know that the foods you eat can affect your brain function on a minute-to-minute basis. If you've ever munched on chips, cookies, or doughnuts and then felt lethargic and unable to focus for the next few hours, you understand how the food-brain connection works. The good news is that eating protein, instead of junk food, provides a number of benefits for the gray matter between your ears.

One of the brain benefits of eating protein is an improvement in both alertness and concentration. Here's how it happens. When you eat protein, it increases levels of tyrosine, an amino acid that spurs the brain to produce greater amounts of dopamine and norepinephrine. These two neurotransmitters are linked to higher energy levels and a greater attention span. When it comes to losing weight, having better energy gives you the get-up-and-go you need to start and stick with an exercise program, follow through with a healthy eating plan, and maintain focus on your ultimate goal when temptations and distractions threaten to derail your efforts.

These same two neurotransmitters are also involved in regulating moods. When your brain doesn't produce enough of these chemical messengers, there's an increased chance for mood disorders such as depression. And when you find yourself in a blue mood, you're more likely to try to soothe yourself with too much of your favorite comfort foods, like chocolate or potato chips. Drinking my protein SuperCharged Smoothies and eating my whole-food meals will provide adequate protein to stabilize your brain and your moods, so you're less likely to engage in emotional overeating.

There's another very important way that dietary protein affects the brain. After more than 20 years of helping my patients lose weight and keep it off, I've seen firsthand how eating protein increases feelings of fullness and curbs appetite. We're just now beginning to understand the biological mechanisms involved in this. When you consume protein, your body digests it by breaking it down into smaller bits known as peptides. What we're learning, thanks to a recent study appearing in the journal *Cell*, is that these peptides send signals to your brain, which then retransmits those signals to your stomach. When your stomach receives these messages, it releases glucose into the portal vein, the major blood vessel that takes blood from your stomach and intestines and carries it to your liver.

What does this blood vessel have to do with feelings of hunger or fullness? The researchers found that the walls of this vein are lined with something called mu-opioid receptors. Stimulating these receptors stimulates your appetite; blocking the receptors suppresses it. When your gut releases glucose into the portal vein, it effectively blocks the receptors and ultimately curbs your appetite.

Your Protein

For each SuperCharged Smoothie or SuperCharged Soup meal, you will have at least 20 grams of protein from protein powder (page 139) and 300 to 370 calories. For each whole-food meal, you will eat at least 30 grams of protein (page 28) and 450 calories. The calories in the fruits and nonstarchy vegetables do not count toward your total calories in your whole-food meals and snacks.

Eating adequate protein is critical for success on the Age-Defying Diet program. Eating the right kinds of protein is equally important. Lean proteins, such as chicken, fish, and non-fatty meats, will feed your muscles and fuel your metabolism. If you're a vegetarian or a vegan, protein powders, soya products, whole grains, and soya foods (men should avoid soya food or soya products, as explained in chapter 3) will provide you with plenty of protein.

While you'll enjoy satisfying SuperCharged Smoothies, Super-Charged Soups, and whole-food meals, the first thing you need to understand is how to know you're eating the right kind and the right amount of protein. When choosing beef, pork, fish, or poultry, or plant-based protein, each ounce of these protein sources counts toward your protein intake.

Avoid higher-fat protein sources because dietary fats can be a contributing factor to insulin resistance and inflammation, both of which promote weight gain.

Grams of Protein and Calories in Animal- and Plant-Based Protein Sources

	Grams of Protein	Calories
Poultry		
Chicken, dark meat (6 oz. raw)	34	212
Chicken, white meat (6 oz. raw)	39	194
Minced chicken (6 oz. raw)	30	243
Skinless, boneless chicken breast (6 oz. raw)	38	204
Chicken, deli meat, lean, rotisserie seasoned (6 oz.)	30	167
Duck, trimmed (6 oz. raw)	31	230
Minced turkey, fat-free (6 oz. raw)	40	190
Minced turkey, 93% lean (6 oz. raw)	32	255
Minced turkey, 85% lean (6 oz. raw)	29	306
Turkey, breast meat (6 oz. raw)	40	194
Turkey, dark meat (6 oz. raw)	36	184
Turkey breast, deli, low-sodium (6 oz.)	39	197

Beef		
Minced beef, 90% lean (6 oz. raw)	34	299
Minced beef, 95% lean (6 oz. raw)	36	233
Rib-eye roast, trimmed (6 oz. raw)	36	260
Top sirloin, trimmed (6 oz. raw)	39	218
Fillet, trimmed (6 oz. raw)	37	236
Bottom sirloin, trimmed (6 oz. raw)	35	280

	Grams of Protein	Calories
Lamb		
Leg of lamb, trimmed (6 oz. raw)	35	224
Lamb loin (6 oz. raw)	36	203

Pork		
Chops (6 oz. raw)	38	226
Tenderloin (6 oz. raw)	36	185
Minced, 96% lean (6 oz. raw)	36	206

Game		
Bison, ground (6 oz. raw)	32	379
Rabbit (6 oz. raw)	37	194
Venison, loin or top round (6 oz. raw)	51	255

Seafood, Canned		
Tuna, light and water-packed (6 oz.)	33	146
Sardines, oil-packed and drained (6 oz.)	42	354
Salmon, drained (6 oz.)	39	235

Seafood, Fresh		
Trout, bass (6 oz. raw)	32	194
Cod, grouper, halibut, tilapia (6 oz. raw)	32	153
Flounder, sole (6 oz. raw)	21	119

(continued)

	Grams of Protein	Calories
Seafood, Fresh (continued)		
Salmon, herring, swordfish (6 oz. raw)	33	262
Tuna (6 oz. raw)	41	185
Mackerel (6 oz. raw)	32	348
Scallops (bay and sea) (6 oz. raw)	21	117
Shrimp (6 oz. raw)	23	121
Crabmeat (6 oz. raw)	31	148
Lobster (6 oz. raw)	28	131

	Grams of Protein	Calories
Soya Products		
Tofu, firm (6 oz.)	12	105
Tempeh (6 oz.)	32	328

	Grams of Protein	Calories
Egg Products		
1 large egg	6	72
1 large egg white	4	17
Egg substitute, liquid (½ cup)	12	58

Essential Amino Acids: Your Body's Building Blocks

Amino acids are the building blocks of all the proteins in your body. These proteins make up your skin, hair, nails, teeth, bones, blood, vital organs, and muscle tissue. They are vital to the process of preserving muscle tissue, critical for optimum brain function, and essential for rebooting a stalled metabolism. Your body naturally produces some, but not all, of the amino acids necessary for these processes. There are eight amino acids, known as *essential* amino acids, that can only be obtained through the foods you eat or with supplements. Additionally, amino acids can't be stored in your body for future use, so you need to get a daily supply of them for optimum health.

Eating an adequate amount of dietary protein, as you'll be doing on the Age-Defying Diet, is one way to increase the levels of essential amino acids you're getting. But as you get older, your body's ability to synthesize protein may diminish, so you may not be getting enough of the essential amino acids you need even if you're eating the recommended amount of protein. Three amino acids in particular—leucine, arginine, and glutamine—are especially important when you're trying to lose weight over the age of 30.

Leucine

Like all essential amino acids, leucine is a building block for protein that helps prevent muscle loss. What makes leucine such a stand-out among amino acids is that it has the highest capacity for muscle building and can prevent muscle loss. In one trial reported in the journal *Clinical Nutrition*, when the researchers added 4 grams of leucine supplements to participants' breakfasts, lunches, and dinners for two weeks, they found that it enhanced the muscle-building process and improved the body's ability to use dietary protein for muscle tissue growth and repair.

Arginine

This is another amino acid that aids in protein synthesis and promotes both muscle building and muscle recovery. Arginine accomplishes this by providing your body with nitric oxide, a chemical that expands blood vessels and allows more blood and nutrients to be pumped more efficiently to your muscles, boosting their growth and repair. Arginine also eliminates ammonia, a waste by-product of protein synthesis, from the body.

Glutamine

Glutamine, the most common amino acid in the human body involved in protein synthesis, plays a pivotal role in hydrating muscle cells and preventing them from breaking down. Every day, your body goes through a natural cycle of breaking down the proteins in your muscle tissue and then regenerating new protein to rebuild the tissue. Your muscles also break down after vigorous physical activity. Scientists have found that lower levels of glutamine are associated with these breakdowns. Taking glutamine as a supplement prior to a workout has been shown to reduce muscle breakdown and lead to muscle growth. As you now know, having more muscle tissue leads to higher metabolism, which means you will burn more fat.

High-Fiber Foods to Fire Up Metabolism

To recharge your metabolism, you also need to eat foods that are packed with fiber. High-fiber foods, including fruits, vegetables, and whole grains—such as my favorites, amaranth, quinoa, and bulgur—cause positive metabolic effects. Scientists have long known that eating appropriate amounts of these foods reduces blood sugar and insulin levels following meals. Over time, this increases insulin sensitivity and helps re-ignite metabolism. Fiber-rich foods also increase feelings of fullness, so you tend to eat less. We're just beginning to discover that eating high-fiber foods also has a more direct beneficial impact on lean muscle mass and body fat.

High-Fiber Foods Safeguard Your Memory

Your brain relies primarily on glucose—a.k.a. sugar—to function. Glucose comes mainly from the fruits, vegetables, and whole grains you eat, which explains why low-carb diets that severely restrict or eliminate healthy fruits, vegetables, and whole grains may affect short-term memory function. Ingesting too much glucose too quickly, such as when you consume refined carbohydrates like candy, cookies, or sugary sodas, can also lead to "brain fog." Eating too much sugar at one time actually damages the cells in your brain and body. High blood sugar over time may lead to age-related memory problems or even Alzheimer's, which some experts are now referring to as "Type 3 diabetes."

To keep your memory sharp, your brain needs a steady stream of glucose. The high-fiber foods you'll be consuming help you achieve this by slowing the digestion process and providing your brain with the slow and steady supply of glucose it needs.

Your Fiber

You'll be getting plenty of fiber from all of the fruits and vegetables you will be eating. You will also eat ½ cup (cooked) serving of whole grains with whole-food meals. Recipes begin on page 209.

Lower Your Metabolic Age with Fruits and Vegetables

Eating fruits and vegetables can reverse your metabolic aging—both inside and out. As each year passes, laugh lines and frown lines on your face become more prominent. Damage is also occurring at the cellular level. Fortunately, plant-based foods that are high in anti-oxidants have an anti-inflammatory effect and can protect your body from the free radicals that cause metabolic and outward aging.

Since fruits and vegetables are high in dietary fiber, they take a long time to digest, because your body has to work harder. The harder your body works, the more your metabolic rate increases and the more calories you burn. Some fruits and vegetables, such as red and green peppers, citrus fruits, brussels sprouts, and broccoli, are a rich source of vitamin C, which also increases metabolism. At the University of Colorado–Boulder, a team of researchers measured resting metabolism before and after giving participants over the age of 60 injections of vitamin C. After the injections, the participants' resting metabolism jumped by an average of nearly 100 calories per day.

Fruits and vegetables contain phytonutrients, the natural and beneficial chemicals found in foods that give them their color and anti-aging power. When choosing the best fruits and vegetables to eat to reboot your metabolism, think about them in color groups. Eat fruits and vegetables from each color group.

• **Greens:** Asparagus, broccoli, kale, and spinach contain disease-fighting chlorophyll.

• **Blues and purples:** Blackberries, blueberries, red grapes, and plums contain memory-improving anthocyanins.

• **Whites:** Bananas, cauliflower, mushrooms, and onions contain anthoxanthins to promote lower blood pressure and proper cholesterol levels.

• **Oranges and yellows:** Apricots, carrots, oranges, and tangerines are packed with beta-carotene for better immune function and visual health.

• **Reds:** Apples, cherries, berries, and tomatoes contain lycopene, which may help lower your risk for cancer.

Your Vegetable

All fruits and all nonstarchy vegetables get the green light on the Age-Defying Diet. You can eat unlimited amounts of the following vegetables with whole-food meals and for snacks. Enjoy them fresh, frozen, or canned—if canned it must be in water or their own juices. You want the kind that aren't packed in syrup, have no added sugar, and are low in sodium.

Artichokes	Mangetaut
Asparagus	Mushrooms
Aubergine	Mustard greens
Bamboo shoots	Okra
Beans (green, wax, Italian)	Onions
Beetroot	Peppers
Broccoli	Rocket
Brussels sprouts	Swede
Butternut squash	Spinach
Cabbage	Spring greens
Carrots	Spring onion
Cauliflower	Sprouts
Celery	(alfalfa, mung bean, lentil)
Cucumber	Swiss chard
Courgette	Tomatoes
Kale	Turnips
Leeks	Turnip tops
Lettuce	Water chestnuts

Your Fruit

You may eat unlimited amounts of the following fruits fresh, frozen, or canned—if canned it must be in water or their own juices. You want the kind that aren't packed in syrup, have no added sugar, and are low in sodium.

Apples

Bananas

Berries (blueberries, blackberries, raspberries, strawberries)

Cherries

Citrus (clementines, grapefruit, lemons, limes, oranges)

Figs

Grapes

Guavas

Kiwi

Mangoes

Melon

Nectarines

Papayas

Peaches

Pears

Persimmons

Pineapples

Plums

Pomegranates

Watermelon

Your Bean and Starchy Vegetable

Beans and starchy vegetables are limited to ½ cup cooked per day.

Beans (black, black-eyed peas, cannellini, chickpeas or garbanzo, kidney, lima, haricot, pinto, red, and white)

Butternut squash

Corn

Lentils

Peas

Potatoes

Pumpkin

Split peas

Sweet potatoes and yams

Drink to Your Good Health

You may be surprised that drinking alcohol can help you lose weight. In a study appearing in *Archives of Internal Medicine*, researchers tracked the drinking habits and weight gain of more than 19,000 healthy-weight women over an average of 13 years. Contrary to what you may suspect, women who drank no alcohol gained the most weight by the end of the trial. How can a glass of wine or beer help reboot and recharge your metabolism? Alcohol, such as wine, may burn calories through a process called thermogenesis. Alcohol raises the body's temperature, which requires your body to burn calories to produce the heat. In the study mentioned above, women who drank alcohol with a meal also ate fewer calories overall, creating a sort of trifecta for weight loss: They burned more calories to digest the wine, burned more calories to increase body temperature, and consumed fewer calories.

Many people believe that alcohol is all sugar or all carbs. Yes, wine is made from grapes, a fruit that contains natural sugars, and beer is made from grains that have carbohydrates. Thanks to the process of fermentation, though, the sugars in both are converted to alcohol and aren't digested as sugar by the body.

The benefits of light alcohol intake don't stop at weight loss. Mountains of scientific evidence have shown that wine, especially red wine, is rich in antioxidants, such as resveratrol, that promote better heart health and are associated with lower blood pressure and cholesterol levels. Even the American Heart Association recommends drinking one 4-ounce serving of wine per day.

Your Wine or Beer

You have the choice—*it is not required*—to drink up to one 6-ounce glass of wine or 12 ounces of beer *with* your whole-food dinner in place of dessert. Drinking alcohol before you eat will trigger your

(continued)

liver to start metabolizing the alcohol almost immediately rather than burning fat. Drinking on an empty stomach also allows alcohol to enter your bloodstream quickly and travel to your brain, where it reduces activity in the areas associated with controlling your behavior. Drinking before eating can lead to poor decision making, such as having another drink or caving in and eating unhealthy foods that are not part of the Age-Defying Diet program. Don't do it!

Drink Water to Speed Up Your Metabolism

Your metabolism is a series of chemical reactions that are dependent on one another. Drinking plenty of water keeps those chemical reactions moving, speeds up your metabolism, and keeps your body functioning properly. Water has been proven to contribute to your body's ability to burn calories.

Sometimes when you think you're hungry or tired, you're actually just thirsty. A glass of water will often do the trick. Your best bet is to drink water throughout the day; don't wait until you're thirsty. Keep a bottle of water in your car or gym bag or on your desk. Add some lime, lemon, and orange wedges with some mint leaves for a fresh flavor.

Your Water

Women: Drink at least 7 8-oz. glasses of water or other liquids with no calories per day. Men: Drink at least 12 8-oz. glasses of water or other liquids with no calories per day. This includes all SuperCharged Smoothie and SuperCharged Soup days.

Get the Right Fats

While our bodies and brains need some dietary fat to maintain optimum health, most people are eating way too much of it—especially saturated fat, which clogs arteries and causes weight gain. Eating too much fat—butter, cheese, fatty cuts of meat—can disrupt metabolic processes and lower your brain's ability to function at top speed.

Your Dietary Fat

All added fats, including "healthy" fats like olive oil, nuts, non-trans-fat spreads, low-fat salad dressings, low-fat dips and sauces, and low-fat mayonnaise are limited. You can also use the following alternatives:

- Coconut cooking spray: 2-second spray
- Fat-free dips and sauces: 1 to 2 tablespoons
- Fat-free salad dressings: 1 to 2 tablespoons
- Fat-free mayonnaise: 1 to 2 tablespoons

Eat Foods to Promote Hormonal Balance and Avoid Hormonal Imbalances

When you're dealing with the hormonal changes that inevitably come with age, women, in particular, need to know which foods can calm the hormonal storms and which ones should be avoided. For instance, soya can help balance women's hormones, but it's the last thing that men should reach for when they're dealing with age-related hormonal changes. I go into great detail about this in chapter 3, starting on page 41.

Metabolism Boosters Everyone Should Eat

Some foods are super metabolism boosters for both men and women. Be sure to include these while you're on this program.

- **Lean beef:** Lean cuts of beef help optimize the muscle-building process so you can lose fat faster.

- **Fatty fish:** High in omega-3 fatty acids, fish like salmon, mackerel, sardines, and tuna reduce inflammation, minimize aches and pains, and lower the risk for Type 2 diabetes, cancer, and heart disease.

- **Spinach:** This dark-green, leafy vegetable reduces acidity in the body, which helps reduce muscle loss to ward off the metabolism meltdown.

- **Nonfat Greek yogurt:** A good source of protein to preserve muscle mass, which ramps up metabolism, Greek yogurt is rich in calcium to protect bones, and high in probiotics to reduce digestive problems.

- **Green tea:** This health-promoting beverage may boost metabolism, helps fight fatigue, and reduces the risk for serious disease.

Eating the foods specifically recommended on the Age-Defying Diet will drop your metabolic age, balance your hormones, reverse muscle loss, boost your brainpower, and result in the pounds melting away. I've provided SuperCharged Smoothies, SuperCharged Soups, and whole-food meal recipes that are easy to prepare and contain the right amounts of calories, protein, fiber, and other nutrients to make sure you lose weight and keep it off. You can also adapt your own recipes or find more on my website DrApovian.com.

CHAPTER 3

Women and Men:
Individual Metabolic Needs

If you're a woman and you once agreed to buddy-diet with your husband, brother, or adult son, I'm sure you noticed how fast he lost weight, while you struggled to shed just a few pounds. That's because the body compositions—the amount of muscle, bone, and fat—of male and female bodies are significantly different. But there are other factors, such as estrogen in women and testosterone in men, that affect weight loss.

Women

Sixty-year-old Priscilla, mother of four grown children and grandmother of five, came to see me at the recommendation of a friend. Priscilla retired early from her job at an insurance company to take care of her grandchildren during the day while their parents were at work. It was easy for Priscilla to eat properly and exercise regularly at her job, because the company had a wellness program for all employees that included healthy food choices in the cafeteria and a gym open from 6 a.m. to 10 p.m. Caring for and running after three little ones was so exhausting that Priscilla wasn't sure if she could continue to look after them. She had gained 40 pounds since leaving her job four years earlier and ate and snacked on whatever the kids left behind—grilled cheese sandwiches or peanut butter and crackers—with cup after cup of coffee for a caffeine jolt. Priscilla couldn't remember the last time she had been to the gym or taken a yoga class. In addition to being overweight, out of shape, and sleep-deprived, Priscilla had to deal with some of the most debilitating effects of menopause—"brain fog" and tiredness because of constantly waking up from hot flashes and sheet-soaking night sweats. She told me, "I'm so tired and foggy when the kids are dropped off at seven in the morning. I worry that one of these days I won't be as alert as I should be and an accident will happen. I don't want to disappoint my children, who totally depend on me. Somehow I feel that if I could lose some weight and get back to my old self, I'd be a better grandmother and babysitter."

By cycling through the Reboot and Recharge phases, Priscilla lost 45 pounds—an additional 5 along with the 40 she was desperate to lose. "It's amazing! I have so much more energy and keep up with my grandchildren. I quickly learned that following this program means more energy and less weight. I feel so much younger."

How Estrogen Affects Weight

Every day, 6,000 U.S. women enter menopause and thousands more cross over into the hormonal "twilight zone" known as perimenopause. No velvet ropes or VIP passes are required here—this is *not* an exclusive club. Every woman on earth eventually receives an invitation to join the party. At the Nutrition and Weight Management Center at Boston University Medical Center, I constantly see patients who are struggling with menopausal and perimenopausal symptoms, including hot flashes, mood swings, and "brain fog," but it's the weight gain that bothers them the most. I regularly hear, "Listen, Dr. Apovian, I can deal with all of that, just help me get rid of this belly fat!" Yes, menopausal weight gain can be the symptom that's hardest to accept. A 2012 study showed that more than 70 percent of the 53 million baby boomer American women are currently trying to lose weight gained as a result of menopause.

Midlife weight gain—particularly around the midsection—is in part due to the complex relationship between the hormone estrogen and fat cells. While the ovaries produce estrogen starting at puberty, what you may not know is that fat cells also manufacture this hormone. When women reach perimenopause or menopause, the amount of estrogen produced by the ovaries decreases, and fat cells race into action to pick up the slack. Fat cells swell in size—the bigger the fat cells, the more estrogen they can produce.

Unfortunately, fat cells also congregate in the midsection. Scientists believe that an expanding waistline occurs because the fat cells in the abdomen are capable of producing more estrogen than fat cells on the hips or thighs.

Extra weight means extra risks for developing serious health conditions, such as insulin resistance, Type 2 diabetes, cardiovascular disease, and metabolic syndrome. And a bulging belly doesn't discriminate. Even if you've been trim and fit your entire life, you may suddenly find yourself having wrestling matches to zip up your favorite jeans.

Do any of these situations sound like yours? Are you a "Professional Dieter," someone who routinely gains weight, then fasts or goes on an extreme diet to lose some pounds quickly? Or are you the magician whose old tricks just aren't working? Those once reliable strategies of cutting calories and upping your cardio workouts no longer help you maintain your weight. Are you trying relentlessly to get rid of those last 5 pounds? These are just a few of the situations that you may find yourself in with a slow metabolism, but don't despair: The Age-Defying Diet will rejuvenate your metabolism and help you lose the weight for good.

To deal with the debilitating effects—weight gain, hot flashes, night sweats, vaginal dryness, sleep disruption, headaches, mood swings, loss of focus—of menopause caused by the body's decreased production of estrogen and progesterone, many women were once prescribed hormone replacement therapy (HRT)—medications containing those missing female hormones. Then a large study showed that those who took HRT had greater risks of heart disease, stroke, and breast cancer. Consequently, HRT guidelines changed, and doctors now prescribe low doses of HRT only in certain circumstances. You need to take matters of aging and hormones into your own hands and prevent age-related muscle and bone loss.

Priscilla began the Age-Defying Diet and lost 8 pounds during the first week by drinking SuperCharged Smoothies and eating lean protein, unlimited fruits and nonstarchy vegetables, and limited whole grains. No more snacking on the children's leftovers or making herself an extra grilled cheese sandwich—or two. Priscilla also made some personal lifestyle changes and asked that the kids be dropped off and picked up 30 minutes later two days a week, so she could fit in her strength-training exercises.

My Approach

Now that you know how hormones play a factor in weight gain and a slower metabolism, let's talk about what we can do to reverse these issues. My patients have had great success with my version of intermittent fasting, which helps you burn fat and shed pounds quickly.

The key to shedding fat is to follow my smoothie fast for the designated amount of time. And it's not a day in which you're starving like on typical fasting or juicing diets. My SuperCharged Smoothies are filling, delicious, and so easy to make that you might want to live on smoothies forever—but don't! It's just a one-day-a-week luxury. Even better, your smoothie day will be a day to get in some R&R and take care of yourself. On other days, as you'll discover in chapter 7, you'll be enjoying one or two SuperCharged Smoothies a day in addition to whole-food meals, snacks, and desserts.

What Women Should Eat and Avoid

It's well known that certain foods deliver more antioxidants, vitamins, and minerals than others and help protect against disorders and illnesses. Others, such as spicy foods, caffeine, and alcohol can exacerbate the uncomfortable, often embarrassing symptoms of menopause.

Foods Women Should Eat

• **Papaya:** After analyzing the blood of more than 13,000 people, scientists from the University of California–San Francisco found that women who had lower levels of vitamin C were more likely to have gallbladder-related illnesses. Papaya packs about twice the amount of vitamin C as does an equal amount of oranges. One medium papaya contains 180mg of vitamin C and a mere 119 calories.

• **Flaxseed meal (ground flaxseeds):** These tiny, fiber-rich, reddish-brown seeds are rich with estrogen-like compounds called lignans that may serve as a potential weapon against breast cancer. A report delivered at the San Antonio Breast Cancer Symposium clearly showed that adding flaxseeds to the diet of women with breast cancer effectively slowed tumor growth. Flaxseeds themselves are not digestible; they must first be ground. Eat 1 to 2 tablespoons of flaxseed meal per day in your SuperCharged Smoothies. (Don't eat any more than that, because it can have a laxative effect.) Flaxseed meal can be purchased in any health food or grocery store. Store flaxseed meal in the refrigerator, so it doesn't turn rancid. Avoid flaxseed oil—it doesn't contain lignans.

• **Tofu:** Foods high in soya protein—tofu, seitan, tempeh, edamame—can lower cholesterol and may help minimize menopausal hot flashes and strengthen bones. Isoflavones, the plant chemicals in soya beans, have a structure similar to estrogen. As women age, they produce less natural estrogen, and the isoflavones in soya may pick up the slack.

• **Bison:** Iron-deficiency anemia occurs when the body does not take in enough iron and makes fewer red blood cells. Iron is necessary for making red blood cells to carry oxygen to other parts of the body. Anemia leads to fatigue and exhaustion. Due to menstruation, women tend to be more anemic than men. Lean bison meat, now available in supermarkets nationwide, provides plenty of iron and less fat than other cuts of beef. Bison burgers are delicious, but because they are so lean, grill them for less time than beef burgers.

• **Dark, leafy greens:** Kale, spring greens, spinach, and beet and turnip tops may help in the fight against osteoporosis, bone disintegration that occurs with aging. While calcium and vitamin D are known to be good for bones, vitamin K, which is bountiful in dark greens, has also been shown to have a positive effect. Researchers who worked on the famous Nurses' Health Study found that women who ate vitamin-K-rich foods (at least 109mcg) were 30 percent less likely to suffer a hip fracture than those who didn't eat their dark greens.

Foods Women Should Eat to Maintain Hormonal Balance

• **Poultry, fatty fish, and soya proteins:** All of these protein sources do more than just help you maintain lean tissue. Research has found that menopausal women lose more weight when most of their protein comes from these ingredients. Some evidence suggests that consuming soya foods may also help alleviate hot flashes and reduce your risk for breast cancer, heart disease, and osteoporosis. Poultry includes chicken and turkey. Fatty fish, such as salmon, mackerel, and sardines, also protect against blue moods, heart disease, and cancer.

• **Cruciferous vegetables:** Broccoli, cabbage, brussels sprouts, cauliflower, and pak choi may fight excess estrogen to lower the risk for breast cancer. Excess estrogen can occur pre-menopause in women who are overweight or obese.

• **B vitamins:** A lack of foods rich in vitamin B can contribute to the feelings of anxiety and depression that can come with menopause. Consume foods high in the B vitamins, such as whole grains and lean beef.

• **Asparagus, melons, and watercress:** These foods help combat one of the most annoying midlife symptoms: bloating.

Foods Women Should Avoid for Hormonal Balance

• **Sugar:** Brown sugar, white sugar, high-fructose golden syrup—call it by any name, sugar has been shown to exaggerate hormonal symptoms in women. That's why your intake of added sugars will be limited on this program. Another benefit is that cutting out sugar may help alleviate some hormonal balance symptoms. A study in the *Journal of the Academy of Nutrition and Dietetics* on women in their 50s and 60s showed that those who decreased their consumption of desserts and sugar-sweetened beverages lost more weight than those who didn't, both over the short term and up to four years later.

• **Caffeinated beverages:** You can drink coffee and tea with a tablespoon of nonfat or low-fat milk and calorie-free energy drinks as well as diet sodas. Know, however, that caffeinated beverages can trigger hot flashes. If you're struggling with hot flashes or night sweats, cut down on caffeine.

• **Alcohol:** Like caffeine, alcohol can spark hot flashes. Although you can drink one glass of wine or beer with your whole-food dinner in place of dessert each night, just say no to alcohol if you're having hot flashes.

• **High-fat foods:** An Australian study of about 6,000 women found that those who reported eating high amounts of high-fat foods—bacon, french fries, ice cream, cheese—also experienced higher rates of hot flashes. The Age-Defying Diet limits fat intake, which may help keep you feeling cool.

• **Spicy foods:** Hold the hot sauce if you want to minimize hot flashes. Stick with herbs and mild spices to flavor food without turning up the heat.

Men

When Charlie, a 54-year-old writer, came to see me, he was unhappy with the 25 pounds he had gained over the last few years. As a novelist who spent a good chunk of the day sitting in front of his computer, he looked forward to his 5-mile daily runs. He enjoyed getting out of his house and socializing with the guys while watching sports, eating pizza, and drinking beer at a local bar. To lose weight, he began to run longer distances, but his knees couldn't take it and the pounds kept piling on around his middle. He found it hard to get a good night's sleep after late nights watching sports and drinking beer. Charlie, who once prided himself on being a self-starter and being at his computer by 8 a.m., was now struggling to get out of bed by 10 a.m.

Mike, a 35-year-old IT guy, works long hours at a major bank. He eats at least two meals a day in the 24-hour cafeteria or gets snacks from vending machines. Even though there's an on-site gym, he's too tired to go after a long day—and night—at work. No wonder his pant size has gone up three times in the last year. He barely sees his two kids and wife; they are fast asleep by the time he gets home.

Dave is a 47-year-old lawyer at a major Wall Street law firm whose workload is so heavy that he rarely has time to eat anything except sandwiches ordered in from the deli. He often grabs a nap on his sofa when time allows. Dave wins case after case, but he still feels depressed and draggy, and has felt his sex drive dwindle. When Dave won a major case, he took his wife to Paris for a long weekend, but even being in the most romantic city in the world, there wasn't much romance or life in the bedroom.

If any of these situations—weight gain around the middle, sleep problems, exhaustion, and erectile dysfunction—sound familiar to you, know that you are not alone. That's why *The Age-Defying Diet* includes this special section devoted to men.

While part of the problem lies in what you eat and how you exercise, there's a more basic issue at the heart of these symptoms.

Low testosterone (low T) is associated with all sorts of male midlife issues: fatigue, sleeplessness, low libido, erectile dysfunction, weakness, depression, and weight gain.

Although it's called the male hormone, testosterone is produced in both men (in the testes) and women (in the ovaries) starting at puberty. Men, however, produce greater amounts of testosterone than women, which gives them specific male characteristics, such as facial hair, sperm production, deeper voice, and so on. Testosterone is essential for maintaining muscle bulk, adequate levels of red blood cells, bone growth, a sense of well-being, and sexual function. Starting in your mid-40s, your testosterone levels drop by about 1 to 2 percent each year. Since testosterone helps build muscle—and its companion, human growth hormone, burns fat—lower levels cause body fat to accumulate in the midsection.

As in your female counterparts, this buildup of body fat tends to target the midsection.

In men, carrying this extra weight compounds the problems associated with aging. Fat ratchets up the metabolizing of testosterone, meaning the more fat on the body, the more quickly it burns through the testosterone, which is already a hormone slipping away. Extra fat leaches testosterone out of the blood, causing energy and libido to wilt. And that paunch is the worst offender. In men, belly fat has the greatest capacity to convert testosterone to estrogen. You can thank, or rather blame, an enzyme in fat tissue known as aromatase for this action. This "estrogenization" can contribute to an overall softer appearance and a drop in virility, which is not what you're going for!

The muscle loss that comes with age, combined with the natural drop in testosterone, lowers the male body's ability to use insulin and may contribute to insulin resistance. With insulin resistance, your body doesn't use the hormone effectively and your pancreas continues releasing more and more insulin. This leaves you with high levels of insulin, which are associated with weight gain, water retention, and excess belly fat. In essence, insulin resistance compounds the metabolism meltdown that is already occurring as the years pass by.

My Approach

Now that you know how hormones play a factor in weight gain and a slower metabolism, let's talk about what we can do to reverse these issues. My patients have had great success with my version of intermittent fasting. You've already learned that as body fat increases in men, testosterone levels decrease. On the flip side, losing weight is associated with an increase in the hormone. My form of intermittent fasting comes into play here, because it helps you burn fat and shed pounds quickly, which pumps up testosterone production.

The key to shedding fat and boosting testosterone is to follow my smoothie fast for the designated amount of time. Many of my male patients think that if one smoothie day a week provides benefits, then smoothie fasting for an entire week must be even better. Sorry, but it doesn't work that way. This is one area in which there can be too much of a good thing. Fasting for longer periods of time can actually decrease testosterone levels. On my program, you cannot have more than one all-smoothie fast day per week to promote healthy testosterone levels. On other days, as you'll discover in chapter 7, you'll be enjoying one or two SuperCharged Smoothies a day in addition to whole-food meals, snacks, and desserts.

When I explain to my male patients how muscle loss affects weight, many of them ask whether testosterone supplements might help reverse the problem. This comes as no surprise, considering how many bodybuilding and men's magazines and websites point to testosterone as a way to bulk up with more muscle. That's when I have to remind them about the potential dangers of hormone therapy. A study on testosterone treatment in older men found that any increases in muscle mass were offset by a rise in cardiovascular disease and heart attacks. The risk was considered so great that this trial was halted early. I then tell them that with the Age-Defying Diet, they will need no pharmaceutical intervention to build muscles and increase testosterone levels. They like that.

Foods Men Should Eat to Increase Testosterone Levels

- **Egg yolks:** Egg yolks may promote increased testosterone levels. If you don't have high cholesterol levels, eat whole eggs a few times each week.

- **Zinc:** Legend has it that oysters are an aphrodisiac, and science may agree. Just two to three oysters deliver a day's supply of zinc, a mineral essential for a well-functioning male reproductive system. Scientists are divided over reports that sperm counts have declined over the last 50 years and that environmental factors are to blame. Research, however, indicates that when men reduce their intake of zinc-rich foods, their testosterone levels fall significantly. Getting adequate zinc is sometimes the answer (11mg per day is recommended for men; more than 40mg can pose risks). In one trial, 22 men with low testosterone levels and sperm counts were given zinc every day for 45 to 50 days. Testosterone levels and sperm counts rose. Since it's unlikely that you'll be eating oysters every day, include other sources of zinc—lean meats, seafood, spinach, and mushrooms—in your diet to protect yourself against prostate cancer, maintain testosterone levels, and enhance sexual function.

- **Whole grains:** Amaranth, barley, quinoa, brown rice, bulgur, and couscous contain vitamins, minerals, and phytochemicals that promote prostate health without wreaking havoc on your metabolism. The trick is to eat small amounts—½ cup of cooked grains with whole-food meals.

Other Foods Men Should Eat

- **Tomato sauce:** When scientists at Harvard University studied what 47,000 male health professionals ate, they found those who ate tomato sauce two to four times per week had a 35 percent lower risk of developing prostate cancer than men who ate none. Lycopene, a phytochemical found in tomatoes, appeared to be responsible.

Research has shown that people—men and women—who eat tomatoes have a lower risk of cancer. Raw tomatoes or tomato juice don't provide protection, however; for lycopene in tomatoes to be absorbed by the body, the tomatoes must be cooked with some kind of fat. Spoon some tomato sauce cooked with a bit of olive oil over a small serving of whole wheat pasta, brown rice, or other grain.

• **Broccoli:** Eating cruciferous vegetables—broccoli, cauliflower, cabbage, and brussels sprouts—may help in the fight against bladder cancer. Bladder cancer, which is common in North America, affects two to three times as many men as women. Researchers who examined the diets of almost 50,000 men discovered that those who ate five or more servings weekly of cruciferous vegetables were half as likely to develop bladder cancer over a 10-year period as men who rarely ate them.

• **Watermelon:** Until the age of 55, men suffer from high blood pressure more than women do. Science has shown that foods rich in potassium can definitively reduce the risk of high blood pressure and stroke. The research convinced the Food and Drug Administration to allow food labels to bear a health claim about the connection between potassium-rich foods and blood pressure. Watermelon, a rich source of this mineral, has more potassium—664mg—in one large slice than the amount found in a banana or a cup of orange juice.

Foods Men Should Limit or Avoid

• **Soya:** It's best to avoid soya foods—tofu, soya milk, edamame, and tempeh—because overconsumption of soya-based foods, with their phytoestrogen-like properties, may cause the male body to develop female attributes, such as enlarged breasts and loss of body hair. In addition, eating a soya-rich diet has been shown to cause sexual dysfunction and contribute to a lack of sexual desire in men.

- **Sugar:** After you eat sugar, your testosterone levels drop, so it's best to avoid sugars in any form, except for those found in fresh fruits and vegetables. Processed sugars are hidden in tens of thousands of products, from fruit juices to snack foods. Even some brands of yogurt as well as savory snacks like potato chips and pretzels contain sugar.

I started Charlie, Mike, and Dave on a regimen of smoothies and healthy whole-food meals, which has been shown to increase levels of certain hormones that trigger the production of testosterone. I stressed how important it was for each of them to find time to exercise with weights to build muscle as well as to work out for cardiovascular health and get a solid night's sleep. Charlie's energy levels are back and he's at his desk at 8 a.m. every day. Those 25 pounds and those late nights at the sports bar are long gone. Mike makes time for short weight-training sessions at his gym and has smoothies at work. Dave also blends his smoothies in the office and makes healthy choices when dining out with clients.

Bottom line? Following the Age-Defying Diet by drinking Super-Charged Smoothies, eating whole foods, and exercising properly and efficiently can help you look younger and feel stronger, while you lose those extra pounds.

CHAPTER 4

The Age-Defying Diet

Now that you're ready to jump-start your metabolism to lose weight for good and feel younger, it's time to talk about the diet. For easy reference, I've included handy symbols—a drinking glass for Super-Charged Smoothies, a bowl for SuperCharged Soups, and a place setting for whole-food meals—to help you keep track of what to eat and drink and when. On the Age-Defying Diet you'll never stress about counting calories or points, or be at a loss over what meals to make. I do the work for you so you can rest assured that what you're eating will keep you fit and get that stubborn metabolism moving!

The Age-Defying Diet has evolved from the medically supervised diet that thousands of my patients have successfully followed to lose hundreds of thousands of pounds. Now you can use this same diet at home.

The Three Steps of the Age-Defying Diet

1. **Reboot—week 1:** Designed to kick your metabolism into high gear by using my version of intermittent fasting, which has proven more effective than traditional diets. This happens with the generous, delicious, filling smoothies you drink, and appetizing and easy whole-food meals.
2. **Recharge—weeks 2 and 3:** Keeps your metabolism revving with the right foods to fuel your body and your brain.

3. **Revitalize—your new lifestyle:** Maintains your metabolism and keeps it working effectively so you remain lean and healthy, and feel younger than your chronological age.

Here's a quick explanation of what you'll be eating and when on the Age-Defying Diet. I've included a day-by-day chart for easy reference and you can find measurement coversion charts in the back of the book (see page 297). Your day-by-day meal plan appears in chapter 7 (page 109). I've done all the work for you so you don't have to waste time figuring out if you're getting enough calories as well as protein and fiber at each meal. The SuperCharged Smoothies and SuperCharged Soups, whole-food meals, and ready-made whole-food meals (page 209) provide you with all the calories and nutrition you need to lose weight and feel younger. Here's what you'll be getting in every recipe: SuperCharged Smoothies and Super-Charged Soups, homemade or instant: 325 to 370 calories; at least 20 grams of protein; 10 grams of fiber. Whole-food meals (includes entrée, side dish, and dessert or optional alcoholic beverage): up to 650 calories; 30 to 45 grams of protein; at least 10 grams of fiber. This nutritional information doesn't include your unlimited fruits and the nonstarchy vegetables that you have with your whole-food meals.

Reboot—Week 1

	Breakfast	Lunch	Snack	Dinner
Day 1		or		or
Day 2		or		plus or

(continued)

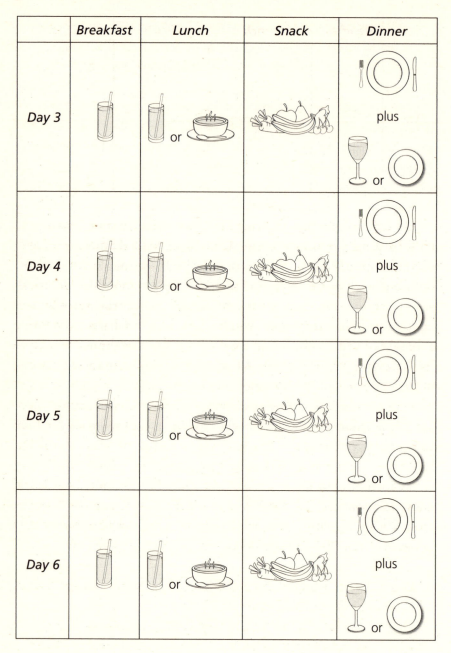

	Breakfast	Lunch	Snack	Dinner
Day 3		or		plus or
Day 4		or		plus or
Day 5		or		plus or
Day 6		or		plus or

	Breakfast	Lunch	Snack	Dinner
Day 7		or		plus or

On day 1 of the Age-Defying Diet, you will give your metabolism CPR by drinking three protein-rich SuperCharged Smoothies (page 138) or SuperCharged Soups (page 191) for your meals. My patients can't believe how delicious and satisfying these smoothies and soups are. What surprises them most is that they have no cravings or hunger pangs. On days 2 through 7, you'll drink a SuperCharged Smoothie at breakfast and lunch and eat a whole-food meal at dinner. (Feel free to switch your smoothie meal from lunch to dinner and/or eat one of the soups instead of any smoothie.)

Dinner might be grilled-to-perfection wild salmon with sautéed spinach and amaranth (a gluten-free whole grain that has more protein than just about any other grain), or a juicy turkey burger on a bed of leafy lettuce and sliced tomatoes with steamed mangetout and brown rice. Every whole-food meal includes: lean protein (page 28), unlimited salads and nonstarchy vegetables (page 35), unlimited fruits, ½ cup cooked grain (page 256), and, with dinner only, 6 ounces of wine or 12 ounces of beer or dessert (page 264). Easy-to-follow recipes start on page 209.

Day 1: Drink 1 SuperCharged Smoothie *or* SuperCharged Soup at each of your three meals.
Day 2: Drink 1 SuperCharged Smoothie for breakfast and 1 SuperCharged Smoothie *or* SuperCharged Soup for lunch. Eat 1 snack of unlimited fruits and nonstarchy vegetables and a whole-food meal for dinner with an optional glass of beer *or* wine *or* dessert.

Day 3: Drink 1 SuperCharged Smoothie for breakfast and 1 SuperCharged Smoothie *or* SuperCharged Soup for lunch. Eat 1 snack of unlimited fruits and nonstarchy vegetables and a whole-food meal for dinner with an optional glass of beer *or* wine *or* dessert.

Day 4: Drink 1 SuperCharged Smoothie for breakfast and 1 SuperCharged Smoothie *or* SuperCharged Soup for lunch. Eat 1 snack of unlimited fruits and nonstarchy vegetables and a whole-food meal for dinner with an optional glass of beer *or* wine *or* dessert.

Day 5: Drink 1 SuperCharged Smoothie for breakfast and 1 SuperCharged Smoothie *or* SuperCharged Soup for lunch. Eat 1 snack of unlimited fruits and nonstarchy vegetables and a whole-food meal for dinner with an optional glass of beer *or* wine *or* dessert.

Day 6: Drink 1 SuperCharged Smoothie for breakfast and 1 SuperCharged Smoothie *or* SuperCharged Soup for lunch. Eat 1 snack of unlimited fruits and nonstarchy vegetables and a whole-food meal for dinner with an optional glass of beer *or* wine *or* dessert.

Day 7: Drink 1 SuperCharged Smoothie for breakfast and 1 SuperCharged Smoothie *or* SuperCharged Soup for lunch. Eat 1 snack of unlimited fruits and nonstarchy vegetables and a whole-food meal for dinner with an optional glass of beer *or* wine *or* dessert.

All 7 days, drink plenty of water or other liquids with no calories.

Recharge—Weeks 2 and 3

	Breakfast	*Lunch*	*Snack*	*Dinner*
Day 8	🥤	🥤 or 🍲		🥤 or 🍲

	Breakfast	Lunch	Snack	Dinner
Day 9				plus or
Day 10		or		plus or
Day 11				plus or
Day 12		or		plus or

(continued)

	Breakfast	Lunch	Snack	Dinner
Day 13				plus or
Day 14		or		plus or

	Breakfast	Lunch	Snack	Dinner
Day 15		or		or
Day 16				plus or
Day 17		or		plus or

	Breakfast	Lunch	Snack	Dinner
Day 18				plus or
Day 19		or		plus or
Day 20				plus or
Day 21		or		plus or

With your metabolism jolted back into action, the next step is to recharge it. For the next two weeks, you'll eat more whole-food meals and lose more weight.

Your next two weeks on the Age-Defying Diet start with another all-smoothies day, followed by alternating days of either two Super-Charged Smoothies and one whole-food meal per day or one Super-Charged Smoothie and two whole-food meals per day. Here's what you'll be eating day by day:

Day 8: Supercharge your day: Have a SuperCharged Smoothie *or* SuperCharged Soup at each of your three meals.

Day 9: Drink 1 SuperCharged Smoothie for breakfast. Eat a whole-food meal for lunch, 1 snack of unlimited fruits and nonstarchy vegetables, and a whole-food meal for dinner with an optional glass of beer *or* wine *or* dessert.

Day 10: Drink 1 SuperCharged Smoothie for breakfast and 1 Super-Charged Smoothie *or* SuperCharged Soup for lunch. Eat 1 snack of unlimited fruits and nonstarchy vegetables and a whole-food meal for dinner with an optional glass of beer *or* wine *or* dessert.

Day 11: Drink 1 SuperCharged Smoothie for breakfast. Eat a whole-food meal for lunch, 1 snack of unlimited fruits and nonstarchy vegetables, and a whole-food meal for dinner with an optional glass of beer *or* wine *or* dessert.

Day 12: Drink 1 SuperCharged Smoothie for breakfast and 1 Super-Charged Smoothie *or* SuperCharged Soup for lunch. Eat 1 snack of unlimited fruits and nonstarchy vegetables and a whole-food meal for dinner with an optional glass of beer *or* wine *or* dessert.

Day 13: Drink 1 SuperCharged Smoothie for breakfast. Eat a whole-food meal for lunch, 1 snack of unlimited fruits and nonstarchy vegetables, and a whole-food meal for dinner with an optional glass of beer *or* wine *or* dessert.

Day 14: Drink 1 SuperCharged Smoothie for breakfast and 1 Super-Charged Smoothie *or* SuperCharged Soup for lunch. Eat 1 snack of unlimited fruits and nonstarchy vegetables and a whole-food meal for dinner with an optional glass of beer *or* wine *or* dessert.

Day 15: Supercharge your day: Have a SuperCharged Smoothie *or* SuperCharged Soup at each of your three meals.

Day 16: Drink 1 SuperCharged Smoothie for breakfast. Eat a whole-food meal for lunch, 1 snack of unlimited fruits and nonstarchy vegetables, and a whole-food meal for dinner with an optional glass of beer *or* wine *or* dessert.

Day 17: Drink 1 SuperCharged Smoothie for breakfast and 1 Super-Charged Smoothie *or* SuperCharged Soup for lunch. Eat 1 snack of unlimited fruits and nonstarchy vegetables and a whole-food meal for dinner with an optional glass of beer *or* wine *or* dessert.

Day 18: Drink 1 SuperCharged Smoothie for breakfast. Eat a whole-food meal for lunch, 1 snack of unlimited fruits and nonstarchy vegetables, and a whole-food meal for dinner with an optional glass of beer *or* wine *or* dessert.

Day 19: Drink 1 SuperCharged Smoothie for breakfast and 1 Super-Charged Smoothie *or* SuperCharged Soup for lunch. Eat 1 snack of unlimited fruits and nonstarchy vegetables and a whole-food meal for dinner with an optional glass of beer *or* wine *or* dessert.

Day 20: Drink 1 SuperCharged Smoothie for breakfast. Eat a whole-food meal for lunch. Eat 1 snack of unlimited fruits and nonstarchy vegetables and a whole-food meal for dinner with an optional glass of beer *or* wine *or* dessert.

Day 21: Drink 1 SuperCharged Smoothie for breakfast and 1 Super-Charged Smoothie *or* SuperCharged Soup for lunch. Eat 1 snack of unlimited fruits and nonstarchy vegetables and a whole-food meal for dinner with an optional glass of beer *or* wine *or* dessert.

All 14 days, drink plenty of water or other liquids with no calories.

If you have reached your weight goal, congratulations! You can move on to Revitalize to maintain your well-earned success. If at the end of Day 21, you want to lose more weight—since everyone loses weight at a different rate and has different amounts of weight to lose—repeat Reboot and Recharge until you reach your goal weight. Then move on to Revitalize.

REVITALIZE

Maintain Your Weight Loss

	Breakfast	Lunch	Snack	Dinner
Day 22	🥤	🥤 or 🍲		🥤 or 🍲
Day 23	🥤	🍽️	🥗	🍽️ plus 🍷 or 🍽️
Day 24	🥤	🍽️	🥗	🍽️ plus 🍷 or 🍽️
Day 25	🥤	🍽️	🥗	🍽️ plus 🍷 or 🍽️

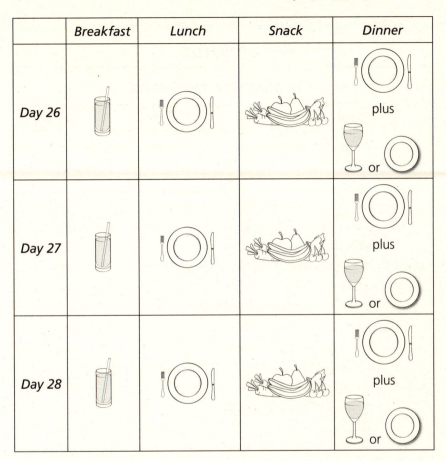

	Breakfast	Lunch	Snack	Dinner
Day 26				plus or
Day 27				plus or
Day 28				plus or

In this final Revitalize phase of the program, you'll have one all-smoothie-or-soup day per week. On the remaining days of the week, you'll drink a SuperCharged Smoothie for breakfast, eat whole-food meals for lunch and dinner, and have one snack of unlimited fruits and nonstarchy vegetables. If you prefer, you can have a whole-food meal for breakfast or lunch, and drink smoothies for lunch or dinner.

Day 22: Drink 1 SuperCharged Smoothie *or* SuperCharged Soup at each of your three meals.

Day 23: Drink 1 SuperCharged Smoothie for breakfast and have a whole-food meal for lunch. Eat 1 snack of unlimited fruits and nonstarchy vegetables, and eat a whole-food meal for dinner with an optional glass of beer *or* wine *or* dessert.

Day 24: Drink 1 SuperCharged Smoothie for breakfast and have a whole-food meal for lunch. Eat 1 snack of unlimited fruits and nonstarchy vegetables, and eat a whole-food meal for dinner with an optional glass of beer *or* wine *or* dessert.

Day 25: Drink 1 SuperCharged Smoothie for breakfast and have a whole-food meal for lunch. Eat 1 snack of unlimited fruits and nonstarchy vegetables, and eat a whole-food meal for dinner with an optional glass of beer *or* wine *or* dessert.

Day 26: Drink 1 SuperCharged Smoothie for breakfast and have a whole-food meal for lunch. Eat 1 snack of unlimited fruits and nonstarchy vegetables, and eat a whole-food meal for dinner with an optional glass of beer *or* wine *or* dessert.

Day 27: Drink 1 SuperCharged Smoothie for breakfast and have a whole-food meal for lunch. Eat 1 snack of unlimited fruits and nonstarchy vegetables, and eat a whole-food meal for dinner with an optional glass of beer *or* wine *or* dessert.

Day 28: Drink 1 SuperCharged Smoothie for breakfast and have a whole-food meal for lunch. Eat 1 snack of unlimited fruits and nonstarchy vegetables, and eat a whole-food meal for dinner with an optional glass of beer *or* wine *or* dessert.

All 7 days, drink plenty of water or other liquids with no calories.

That's the Age-Defying Diet. It couldn't be easier to follow, and you will be astonished by the results you get in just three weeks' time. And remember, you're not on your own when it comes to recipes and meal plans—just turn to chapter 7 for meal plans and to chapters 8 through 10 for recipes, and if you would like more recipes with your favorite foods, sign up for the online Age-Defying Coach. Signing up is free with this book (see page 294). I know you can succeed on my diet. My readers are as important to me as my patients. If you have questions, concerns, or difficulties, don't hesitate to contact me on Facebook, Google Plus, Pinterest, Twitter, or through my website DrApovian.com. I am here to help you.

CHAPTER 5

The Age-Defying Workout

On my program you will be doing exercises only two days a week, and for only nine minutes up to thirty minutes—that's all you do. These are strength training exercises, but not strength training exercises that will bulk you up like a bodybuilder. With these timesaving workouts you will not only lose weight but make your body lean and firm. My exercise programs—I offer you a choice—will keep you from dropping muscle along with the fat while speeding up your metabolism. They will also supercharge your energy, improve your moods, sharpen your brain, and even add years to your life.

Strength Training Burns More Fat and Calories than Other Exercises

Of the thousands of people who have come to me for help losing weight, not one of them has ever asked, "Can you help me gain more metabolically active tissue?" Instead, they all arrive in my office with the same request: "Help me lose all this fat." What I help them understand is that in order to lose that extra fat around the midsection they have to build up their muscles. As previously explained, muscle burns seven times more calories than fat. The more lean muscle you have, the more efficiently your body will burn the calories you take in. Don't worry; you don't have to become a bodybuilder or an Olympian to gain the benefits. With my program, you will gain the muscle that you need to lose weight and look fit and toned.

The best way to develop lean tissue to boost your metabolism and burn more calories is with strength training, also known as resistance training. Until recently, it was seen as exercise that only bodybuilders, professional athletes, and Olympians performed as part of their training routines. There was no reason for the general population to engage in such activities. When we became more sedentary—spending long hours at a desk or on a couch, in front of a computer or a TV—it was recommended that we get at least 30 minutes of cardiovascular exercise at least five times per week. Many reasoned that spending at least double that amount of time on a treadmill, stair climber, bicycle, or elliptical would be even more beneficial.

Cardiovascular workouts are great for heart-lung health, but they offer little, if any, benefit when it comes to sarcopenia, the loss of muscle that is replaced by fat. The best way to burn fat and fight muscle loss is with a protein-rich diet and strength training combined with some cardio exercise.

If you go on a traditional diet and work out like a hamster on a wheel, you will lose fat as well as muscle. The results? You become thinner, but you also become soft and pudgy.

According to Quincy College's exercise scientist Wayne West-cott, PhD, my exercise consultant for the Age-Defying Diet, the benefits of resistance training include:

> Improved physical performance, movement control, walking speed, functional independence, cognitive abilities, and self-esteem. Resistance training may also assist in prevention and management of Type 2 diabetes by decreasing visceral fat... and improving insulin sensitivity. Resistance training may enhance cardiovascular health, by reducing resting blood pressure, decreasing the "bad" cholesterol and triglycerides, while increasing the "good" cholesterol. Resistance training may promote bone development with studies showing 1 percent to

3 percent increase in bone mineral density. Resistance training may be effective for reducing low back pain and easing discomfort associated with arthritis and fibromyalgia and has been shown to reverse specific aging factors in skeletal muscle.

Lift Weights...and Your Metabolic Rate

Inactive adults experience a 3 to 8 percent loss of muscle mass per decade. Ten weeks of strength training has been shown to increase the metabolic rate in formerly inactive adults by 7 percent and boost daily calorie expenditure by 15 percent.

Without a doubt, strength training is the best way to develop metabolically active muscle tissue, which is the most efficient way to facilitate fat loss. Experts agree that if you aren't lifting weights already, then start now. By engaging in a strength-training program, your body will ignite your metabolism into fat-burning mode. For decades, the American College of Sports Medicine (ACSM) has been investigating the role of strength training as a means to boost metabolism and increase fat burning. In one study published by ACSM, a total of 1,644 adults between the ages of 21 and 80 completed a 10-week training program that involved either two or three workouts a week. On average, people ages 45 to 54 added 3.1 pounds of lean muscle while those younger than that added 2.5 pounds of muscle. Even better, training just two days a week was as effective as doing it three times per week.

In the same study, participants across all age groups not only gained lean tissue but also lost an average of approximately 4 pounds of body fat in the same amount of time. For the group between the ages of 45 and 54 who gained just over 3 pounds of lean muscle, that means there was basically a 7-pound switcheroo in the fat-to-lean tissue ratio, effectively reversing the metabolism meltdown. If strength training alone provides that much of a metabolic turnaround, think how much better your results will be when you combine strength training with the proven eating plan and other strategies detailed in this book!

It's important to understand that strength training doesn't mean bodybuilding or bulking up. Women, in particular, are concerned that if they lift weights, they will look like bulky bodybuilders. That can't happen. Bodybuilders are bulky because they have favorable genetics, spend hours every day lifting heavy amounts of weight, and eat a specific diet geared to pumping up their muscle mass. With the Age-Defying Workout, you'll be lifting light weights just twice a week. You'll create the lean, toned body you want, not an overly muscular one.

To give you an idea of how effective strength training and nutrition are, look at the results of a study that Dr. Westcott, a team of scientists, and I did. We compared the effects of exercise alone versus exercise combined with specific nutrition programs on body composition and blood pressure. We enlisted 99 women and 22 men between the ages of 20 and 86 for the trial and placed them in one of three groups:

1. **Exercise Only:** These participants followed a strength and endurance program with no changes in what they ate.
2. **Exercise/Protein:** These volunteers followed the same exercise regimen in addition to meeting a daily protein requirement.
3. **Exercise/Protein/Diet:** This group followed an identical protocol as the Exercise/Protein group but restricted daily caloric intake to 1,200 to 1,500 calories for women and 1,500 to 1,800 calories for men.

After 10 weeks, the Exercise/Protein group (2) lost more weight and inches than the Exercise Only (1) group. The Exercise/Protein/Diet group (3) lost even more weight and inches than the other two groups.

These findings suggest that combining exercise with a higher-protein diet, such as the Age-Defying Diet, will enhance the effects of exercise, keep you healthy, and help you lose more weight, shed more fat, shrink your waist, and increase lean muscle mass.

In another study, researchers tested the effects of a low-calorie diet alone versus a high-protein diet plus resistance training. After 12 weeks, the low-calorie-diet group lost just 5.5 pounds of body fat while the people who followed the high-protein diet and did resistance training lost more than 15 pounds of body fat. Note that this was just the amount of *body fat* they lost, not their total weight loss. Depending on your height, losing 15 pounds of body fat without sacrificing lean tissue could mean dropping a dress size for women or 4 inches in pant size for men.

So What About That Cardio Workout?

The *only* exercise that will reboot your metabolism and lead to permanent weight loss is strength training. As you now know, when you lose muscle, your metabolism is compromised and doesn't function at its best. There are only two ways to gain muscle and reboot your metabolism: Change what you eat and exercise with weights.

If you've been running on a treadmill or spinning on a bicycle for hours while eating a low-calorie diet to lose weight, then you've been wasting your time. Aerobic, or cardiovascular, exercise burns fat but does not build muscle. I don't want you to give up or avoid your cardio workouts. Aerobic exercise keeps your heart pumping blood effectively, increases your lung capacity, reduces stress, boosts your energy levels, maintains mood levels, and promotes better sleep. Taking a 30-minute walk every day or going to spin class two or three times a week is important. If, however, you want to reboot your metabolism and lose weight, then you also need to pick up those weights.

Put Some Pep in Your Step

When 36-year-old Roberta came to my office, she was 20 pounds overweight, but her biggest complaint wasn't about her weight. "Sure, I'd love to lose these extra pounds and drop a dress size, but the thing that drives me crazy is that I just don't have the energy I used to have. I can barely get out of bed at seven in the morning and get to work on time. By late afternoon, I want to put my head down on my desk and take a nap. What's really odd is that I seem to get a second wind just before bedtime and can't fall asleep until one thirty or two o'clock. Then the whole cycle starts over again."

New patients frequently tell me how tired they are and wonder why they feel so sluggish. "Why don't I have the energy I once did?" As I've explained, metabolic aging causes everything in your body and brain to slow down.

The Age-Defying Workout will give you the energy boost you've been craving. One way that strength training boosts your energy levels is by increasing the body's production of AMP kinase, a metabolic enzyme that provides cellular energy. When your cells contain more energy, you have more energy. Physical activity of any kind boosts production of AMP kinase, which ultimately puts a little more pep in your step and gives you the energy you need to get off the couch and move more. Increased amounts of AMP kinase give you more energy throughout the day and minimize fatigue.

One of my research studies showed that AMP kinase is lower in obese people who are insulin-resistant than in obese people who are insulin-sensitive. What this boils down to is that AMP kinase increases after weight loss, which means that as you lose weight on the Age-Defying Diet, you will begin to feel younger and more energetic.

After nine weeks of drinking smoothies, eating whole-food meals, and lifting weights for the first time, Roberta lost 25 pounds and 7 inches around her waist. She was actually able to wear pants and skirts that were hidden in the back of her closet, because she was leaner and thinner thanks to the Age-Defying Diet. Most of all, Roberta says she now falls asleep when her head hits the pillow and is out of bed before her alarm goes off in the morning.

Other Benefits of Strength Training

Lower Your Stress Levels

In today's busy world, there's no escaping stress—and that's bad news for your body *and* your belly. Whether it's work, caring for children and parents, or financial worries, there are plenty of stressful situations that assault us every day.

What does this mean for your waistline? Research shows that stress and fat feed off each other in a vicious cycle. When you're under chronic stress, your body releases more of the stress hormone cortisol. People who are overweight or obese tend to have higher levels of cortisol. Stress makes it harder for men to lose that spare tire because high levels of cortisol have been found to block the effectiveness of testosterone.

The Age-Defying Workout strength-training program is the best way to lower your cortisol and stress levels. In general, people who are more physically fit tend to have lower levels of stress hormones than those who are couch potatoes. Having more muscle mass can help you cope with stressful situations—as researchers at the Medical College of Georgia found when they tested how people's blood pressure recovered after stress. Typically, when you're under stress, your blood pressure rises. After the stressful situation has passed, your blood pressure should come back down. In people with higher percentages of lean body mass, their blood pressure returned to normal sooner.

Sharpen Your Brain

Emerging evidence shows that strength training can actually make you smarter. Brazilian researchers conducted studies on rats to evaluate the brain benefits of strength training and aerobic exercise. One group of rats did a form of "weight lifting." To simulate resistance training, the researchers attached a weight to the rats' tails for training sessions over an eight-week period. Another group of rats ran on a treadmill, and a third group did nothing. At the end of the trial, the weight-lifting rats and the running rats had increased levels of BDNF, the protein that helps your brain generate new neurons. These two groups of rats also performed at high levels on tests of learning and memory. In essence, the rats became smarter with exercise.

These results don't come as a surprise to Teresa Liu-Ambrose, a researcher at the Brain Research Center of the University of British Columbia, who has long studied the effects of strength training on people. One of her trials, which appeared in an issue of *PLoS One*, involved older women who were experiencing signs of memory loss. Her findings showed that among these women, those who lifted weights performed better on cognitive tests than did the women who completed low-intensity exercises such as arm circles or leg lifts without resistance or weights.

Your brain gets in on the act in other ways, too. Much has been written about how cardiovascular exercise, such as running or cycling, can be a real mood booster because it enhances production of the body's natural, feel-good neurochemical endorphin. What you may not know is that strength training can also brighten moods, reduce anger and irritability, and improve self-esteem. I see it all the time in my patients. As they progress through the program, they become happier and more self-confident.

Build Up to Bone Up

Osteoporosis is a disease that occurs when bones lose their density due to decreased amounts of calcium and other minerals, and broken bones can be the result. As you get older, osteoporosis becomes a greater risk: With each passing year you're more likely to lose bone density and develop weak, brittle bones. For women, as hormone levels fall during perimenopause and menopause, the risk for thinning bones becomes even greater. Statistics show that 50 percent of all women will break a bone due to osteoporosis. Men over the age of

50 are more likely to suffer a bone break caused by osteoporosis than to get prostate cancer.

Studies have repeatedly shown that strength training helps prevent bone loss and may even build new bone. Some studies have shown that following a strength-training program can produce significant increases in a woman's bone density, so if you already have osteoporosis, a strength-training regimen may help.

Don't Just Live Longer, Live Better!

Resistance training has been found to reduce the risk for myriad debilitating diseases, including Type 2 diabetes, cancer, high blood pressure, and heart disease.

Australian scientists found that people with Type 2 diabetes who engaged in a progressive resistance-training program (meaning they gradually increased the amount of weight they lifted) three days a week reduced their insulin resistance and improved their blood sugar control. The researchers noted that the improvements in metabolic health were similar to those seen when adding a second diabetes medication. Lifting weights may also help prevent the onset of Type 2 diabetes thanks to improved insulin sensitivity, which makes it easier for your body to shuttle sugar out of your bloodstream and into the cells of your metabolically active muscles.

My exercise program can also protect you from the cellular damage caused by free radicals associated with cancer, cardiovascular disease, and other diseases. Scientists found that people who did resistance training three times a week for six months had significantly less oxidative cell damage than those who didn't lift weights. Another team of researchers shared their findings that resistance training may reduce the risk for colon cancer. When it comes to cancer, strength training can be particularly protective for men. Researchers found that men with higher muscle strength are up to 40 percent less likely to die from cancer.

My exercise program can also lower your blood pressure, which protects your heart and reduces your risk of stroke. And if you do develop a serious condition, such as cardiovascular disease or cancer, doing strength training is essential. A team of researchers examined all the existing scientific findings on muscle strength and health and concluded that the more muscularly fit you are, the less likely you are to die from heart disease, cancer, and certain other diseases.

You're Never Too Old to Start Exercising

Easing into my program, regardless of your age, will help reverse many of the conditions that are the cause of your metabolism meltdown. Many people feel self-conscious or nervous about getting back into an active lifestyle but the fact is, being active is the key to preventing serious disease and weight gain. Regular exercise also keeps your body and brain full of healthy hormones that will keep your moods uplifted.

By gradually increasing the amount of weight you lift and sticking with my program, you will ensure that your metabolism gets you back to a younger, stronger, thinner you.

The Age-Defying Workout

The Age-Defying Workout focuses on strength-training moves that work the major muscle groups in your body to give your metabolism the biggest boost possible. Even if you've never lifted weights before, you'll be able to do this quick and effective routine. This is the surefire way you'll be increasing your metabolism.

Like most of my patients, you're no doubt busy and don't have hours to dedicate to a workout routine. That's why this workout program has been engineered to provide maximum results in the least amount of time possible. With this routine, you'll be doing compound exercises, which means you'll be working more than one group of muscles at a time. You'll get a total-body workout in a short amount of time. In one single move, you may be working your thighs, butt, core, shoulders, and back—all at the same time! That's what I call efficient. It's a routine that can fit into the busiest lifestyle, whether you're raising kids, caring for your aging parents, holding a high-level position at work, or all of the above.

The Age-Defying Workout instructs you to lift weights for a specific amount of time. In contrast, traditional workout routines tell you to lift weights a specific number of times (reps) and then repeat that number several times (sets). In this program, you'll be alternating the exercises as many times as you can within a one-minute window. Working quickly for this amount of time works your muscles and gets your heart pumping. To get the most out of these exercises, think quality not quantity. It's not the number of repetitions you do that matters, but rather maintaining proper form and going through the full range of motion with each repetition.

These exercises are also geared to work with the Age-Defying eating plan and ensure that you're working out at the optimum level during each phase. During the Reboot phase, you'll be doing only two exercises for a total of just nine minutes twice a week. In the Recharge phase, you'll do 18 minutes twice a week, and in the Revitalize phase only 30 minutes twice a week. Somewhere along the line, we've been taught to think that the more we work out, the better our bodies will be. That's not true. To get the greatest benefits from my program, you never need to perform the exercises more than two times a week for 30 minutes.

Here's the big secret of strength training: Once you get into a strength-training routine, your body continues to burn fat for up to 48 hours after your workout session!

Strength Training Tips

- If you've never used weights before, don't worry. When you begin, start with light weights, or even no weights, and gradually progress to heavier ones. The goal is to lift those weights until you can't lift them anymore. As you near the end

(continued)

of each 60-second period, the last few repetitions should be challenging—almost impossible—for you to complete. If, for example, you can lift 2-pound weights without difficulty, then use 5-pound weights instead. If you can only make it to 30 seconds, then the weights are too heavy. Experiment to find the right amount of weight for your individual fitness level. As you become stronger and you find that the weights you're using are too easy, it's time to go up to the next level.

- Warm up for a few minutes before lifting weights. To warm up, walk in place or on a treadmill. You can also do each of the recommended exercises *without* weights 10 times.
- Keep this book handy so you can easily refer to the exercises.
- When lifting weights, proper form and posture are essential—more important than the amount of weight lifted. Check your form in a mirror as you work out. If you're not sure whether you're doing the exercises properly, then consider taking a weight-training class at a local gym or sign up for the Age-Defying Coach, which comes free with this book (see page 294) for videos and tips from top experts.

Age-Defying Workout

Reboot: 9 minutes, 2 exercises, 2 times a week. With only 2 exercises to follow, this phase is a great way to ease into your Age-Defying Workout routine.

Recharge: 18 minutes, 4 exercises, 2 times a week. Two new exercises are added to your routine in this phase.

Revitalize: 30 minutes, 5 exercises, 2 times a week. One new exercise is added in this phase.

You'll continue with Revitalize to maintain your lean muscle mass and newly acquired shape.

Add More Weight-Bearing Activity Every Day

My exercise workout is what I would like you to be doing on the Age-Defying Diet, but if for some reason you can't, do what you can to increase your weight-bearing activity. Weight-bearing activities are any form of movement in which you must support your own weight. This type of exercise forces your muscles to work against gravity, which increases their strength to fire up metabolism and melt more fat. Examples include taking the stairs instead of the elevator, parking in the farthest spot at the grocery store and carrying the heavy grocery bags all the way across the parking lot, or carrying your toddler rather than pushing him or her in the stroller.

Make an effort to do some sort of weight-bearing exercise every day. The easiest type of weight-bearing exercise? Take a walk! Put on your sneakers, head out the door, tune into some songs on your smartphone, and walk briskly for 30 minutes. Mix up your weight-bearing exercises. While walking is great for hips and legs, yoga is ideal for your arms and back.

The Age-Defying Workout
Using Free Weights

Start with just the following two exercises for the Reboot Phase, then move on to the Recharge and Revitalize exercises. If you have never used weights before, do the exercises without them. Once you feel comfortable with the exercises, then add weights, starting with 1-pound weights and increasing by an additional pound as the previous weights become too easy to lift. The weights you use are less important than performing the exercises for the complete amount of time.

Reboot Phase

Do the following two exercises for nine minutes, twice a week.

- Do as many Squats with Biceps Curls as you can in 60 seconds, then rest for 30 seconds.
- Do as many Lunges with Lateral Raises as you can in 60 seconds, then rest for 30 seconds.
- Repeat until you have done each exercise three times.

Squats with Biceps Curls: Stand with a weight in each hand by your sides. Your feet should be slightly wider than hip distance apart throughout the performance of this exercise (Fig. 1). As you sit down into a squat position, simultaneously curl the weights up toward your shoulders (Fig. 2). As you stand up, lower your arms to your sides. Repeat for 60 seconds.

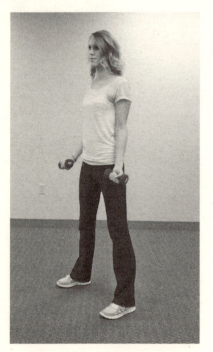
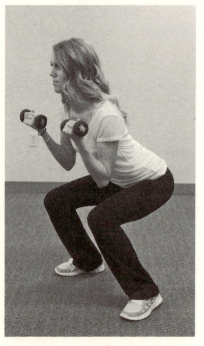

(Fig. 1)   Starting Position   (Fig. 2)   Ending Position

Lunges with Lateral Raises: Stand with a weight in each hand by your sides (Fig. 3). With your left leg, step far enough forward into a lunge so that your knee is in line with your ankle (neither in front of nor behind your ankle). Your front thigh and rear shin should be almost parallel to the floor. Simultaneously, raise both arms parallel to the floor with elbows at a 45-degree angle (Fig. 4). As you push off the left foot to stand up, return your elbows to your sides. Repeat with the left leg. Alternating the right and left legs, repeat for 60 seconds.

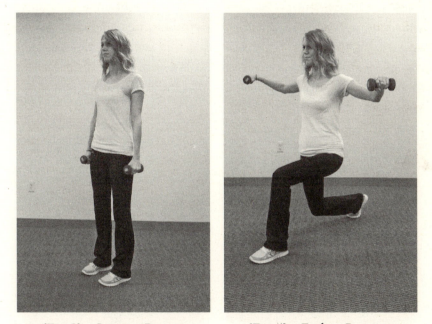

(Fig. 3)   Starting Position   (Fig. 4)   Ending Position

Recharge Phase

Do the following four exercises for 18 minutes, twice a week.

- Do as many Squats with Biceps Curls as you can in 60 seconds, then rest for 30 seconds.
- Do as many Lunges with Lateral Raises as you can in 60 seconds, then rest for 30 seconds.

- Do as many Deadlifts to Upright Rows as you can in 60 seconds, then rest for 30 seconds.
- Do as many Plié Squats with Triceps Extensions as you can in 60 seconds, then rest for 30 seconds.
- Repeat until you have done each exercise three times.

Deadlifts to Upright Rows: Begin in a squat position with a weight in each hand. Keep your head up, shoulders down, and back straight (Fig. 5). As you slowly rise, bring the weights to chest level, keeping them close to your body and leading with your elbows (Fig. 6). Slowly squat back down, lowering the weights toward your feet. Repeat for 60 seconds.

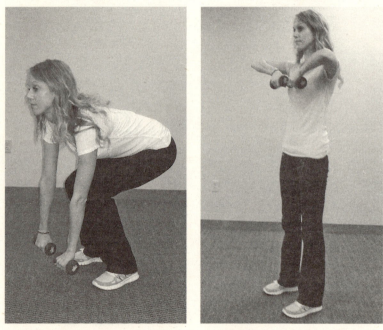

(Fig. 5)   Starting Position   (Fig. 6)   Ending Position

Plié Squats with Triceps Extensions: Stand with a weight in each hand, elbows bent by your sides, feet wider than hip-width apart, toes pointed outward (Fig. 7). As you squat, keep your elbows fixed and extend your arms behind you (Fig. 8). As you straighten your legs, keep your elbows fixed and bring your hands back toward your chest. Repeat for 60 seconds.

Plié Squats with Triceps Extensions

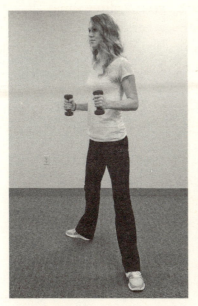 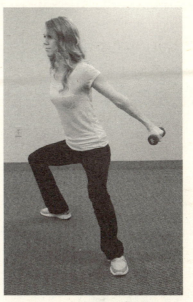

(Fig. 7)   Starting Position   (Fig. 8)   Ending Position

Revitalize Phase

Do the following five exercises for 30 minutes, twice a week.

- Do as many Squats with Biceps Curls as you can in 60 seconds, then rest for 30 seconds.
- Do as many Lunges with Lateral Raises as you can in 60 seconds, then rest for 30 seconds.
- Do as many Deadlifts with Overhead Presses as you can in 60 seconds, then rest for 30 seconds.
- Do as many Plié Squats with Overhead Triceps Extensions as you can in 60 seconds, then rest for 30 seconds.
- Do as many Planks with One-Arm Rows as you can in 60 seconds, then rest for 30 seconds.
- Repeat until you have done each exercise four times.

Deadlifts with Overhead Presses: Begin in a squat position with a weight in each hand (Fig. 9). Keep your head up, shoulders down, and back straight. As you slowly rise, bring your hands up to your shoulders, then press, or raise, the weights directly overhead (Fig. 10). As you slowly squat back down, bring your hands to your shoulders, and then down toward your feet. Repeat for 60 seconds.

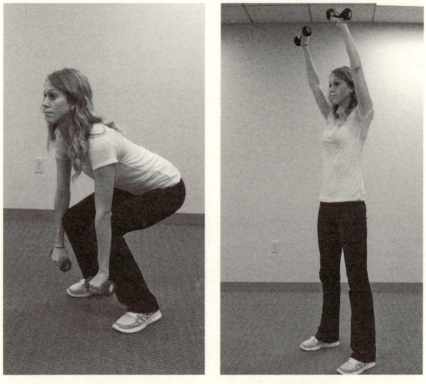

(Fig. 9)   Starting Position   (Fig. 10)   Ending Position

Plié Squats with Overhead Triceps Extensions: Holding a weight in each hand directly above your head (Fig. 11), lower yourself into a squat (keeping your knees in line with your ankles). Then lower the weights behind your head by bending your elbows (Fig. 12). Return to the starting position by pressing through your heels and simultaneously straightening your legs and arms. Repeat for 60 seconds.

Plié Squats with Overhead Triceps Extensions

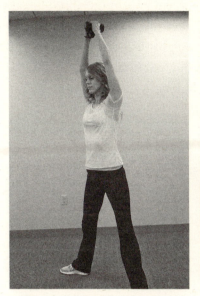
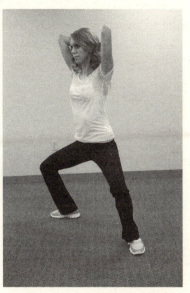

(Fig. 11)   Starting Position   (Fig. 12)   Ending Position

Planks with One-Arm Rows: Hold a weight in each hand against the floor, with your abdominals contracted and your legs extended in a straight line so that you are balanced on your hands and feet (Fig. 13). Holding this straight-body position, bring your left hand/weight toward your shoulder and return to the floor (Fig. 14). Repeat with your right hand/weight, alternating arms for 60 seconds.

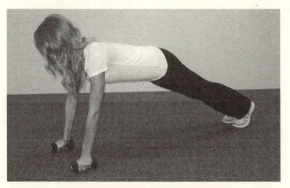

(Fig. 13)   Starting Position

Planks with One-Arm Rows

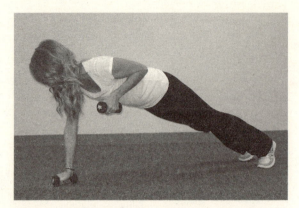

(Fig. 14)   Ending Position

Alternative Exercises Using Weight Machines

If you belong to a gym and prefer to use weight machines instead of free weights, here are the exercises you should do to recharge your metabolism and lose weight. The amount of weight lifted is different for everyone, but here's a simple way to determine how much weight to lift with the machines: The goal is to use weights that are light enough to do at least 10 repetitions but heavy enough so the last 2 reps take some additional effort. If you can do an exercise at least 15 times without any effort, then you need to increase the amount of weight you're using. Start with an increase of 5 or 10 pounds. As you continue to lift weights during the coming weeks and months, you will need to increase the amount you lift to challenge yourself. Be sure to pay close attention to your form.

Reboot Phase—Alternative Exercises Using Weight Machines

Do each of the following two exercises twice a week.

Leg Presses: Adjust the seat so that your legs are bent at 90 degrees when you sit down. With feet, knees, and hips in alignment, place your feet evenly on the footplate and your hands on the handles (Fig. 15). Press the footplate forward until your knees are fully extended (Fig. 16). Slowly lower the weight—don't let the weight drop and slam down—and return to the starting position. Repeat for 60 seconds or at least 10 times.

Leg Presses

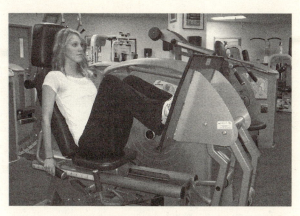

(Fig. 15)   Starting Position

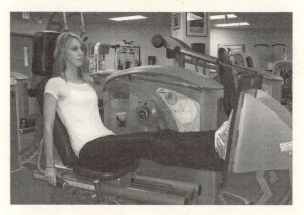

(Fig. 16)   Ending Position

Pull-Downs: Adjust the seat so your hands just reach the bar. Sit upright, with your thighs securely under the pads, hands shoulder-width apart on the bar, and palms facing in (Fig. 17). Pull the bar down to shoulder-height (Fig. 18). Slowly return the handle to the starting position. Repeat for 60 seconds.

Pull-Downs

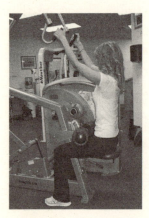 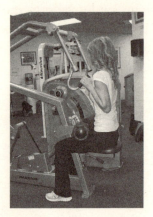

(Fig. 17)   Starting Position   (Fig. 18)   Ending Position

Recharge Phase—Alternative Exercises Using Weight Machines

Do the Leg Presses and Pull-Downs twice a week. In addition, do each of the following two exercises twice a week.

Chest Presses: Sit upright with your chest directly behind the bars. Grasp the handles with your arms parallel to the floor (Fig. 19). Press the handles forward until your elbows are fully extended (Fig. 20). Slowly return to the starting position. Repeat for 60 seconds.

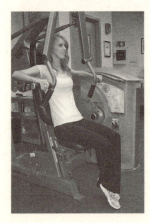 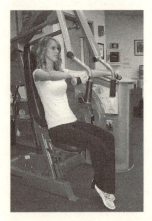

(Fig. 19)   Starting Position   (Fig. 20)   Ending Position

Abdominal Flexions: Sit with your upper back against the pad. Place your ankles behind the rollers and elbows on the arm pads (Fig. 21). Grasp the handles and curl forward until your trunk and hips are fully flexed (Fig. 22). Slowly return to the starting position. Repeat for 60 seconds.

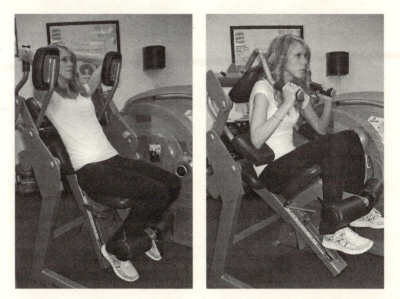

(Fig. 21)   Starting Position   (Fig. 22)   Ending Position

Revitalize Phase—Alternative Exercises Using Weight Machines

Do the Leg Presses, Pull-Downs, Chest Presses, and Abdominal Flexions twice a week. In addition, do the following exercise twice a week.

Rotary Torso: Face forward with your torso erect and your legs gripping the seat extension. Place your upper left arm behind the pad and your right upper arm against the pad (Fig. 23). Rotate your torso 45 degrees to the right (Fig. 24). Slowly return to the starting position. Repeat for 60 seconds. Place your upper right arm behind the pad and your left arm against the pad. Rotate your torso 45 degrees to the left. Slowly return to the starting position. Repeat for 60 seconds.

Rotary Torso

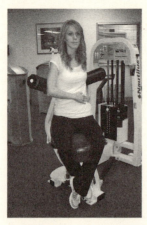
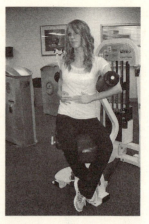

(Fig. 23)   Starting Position   (Fig. 24)   Ending Position

Optional Weight Machine Exercises

If you would like to do additional weight exercises, then add these to your routine once you feel comfortable with the previous exercises.

Shoulder Presses: Sit upright with your shoulders lower than the handles. Grip the handles with your hands (Fig. 25) and press them up until your elbows are fully extended (Fig. 26). Slowly return to the starting position. Repeat for 60 seconds.

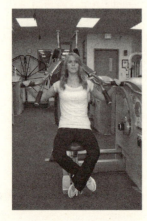
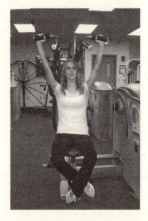

(Fig. 25)   Starting Position   (Fig. 26)   Ending Position

Hip Abductions: Sit with both knees inside the movement pads, your feet on the supports with your legs together, and your hands on the handles (Fig. 27). Using your legs, push the movement pads as far apart as you can (Fig. 28). Slowly return the pads to the starting position. Repeat for 60 seconds.

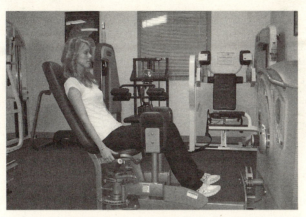

(Fig. 27)   Starting Position

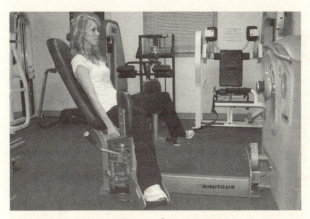

(Fig. 28)   Ending Position

Hip Adductions: Sit with both knees outside the movement pads, your feet on the supports with legs apart, and your hands on the handles (Fig. 29). Using your legs, push the movement pads together (Fig. 30). Slowly return the pads to the starting position. Repeat for 60 seconds.

Hip Adductions

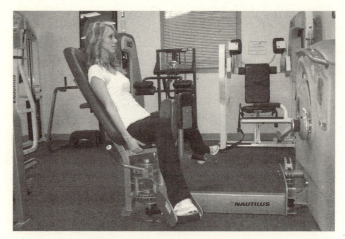

(Fig. 29)   Starting Position

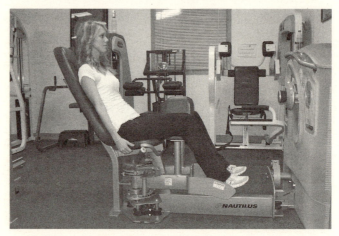

(Fig. 30)   Ending Position

Leg Extensions: Sit with your back against the pad and your knees flexed at approximately 90 degrees, your ankles behind the roller and your hands on the handles (Fig. 31). Lift the roller pad until your knees are fully extended (Fig. 32). Slowly return the pad to the starting position. Repeat for 60 seconds.

Leg Extensions

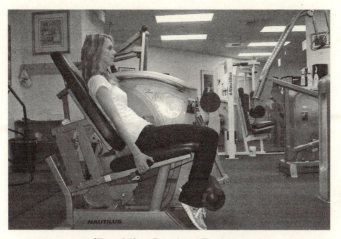

(Fig. 31)   Starting Position

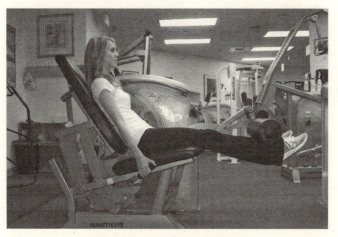

(Fig. 32)   Ending Position

Leg Curls: Sit with your back against the pad, your knees fully extended, your legs between the roller pads, and your hands on the handles (Fig. 33). Pull the roller pads backward until your knees are fully flexed (Fig. 34). Slowly return the pad to the starting position. Repeat for 60 seconds.

Leg Curls

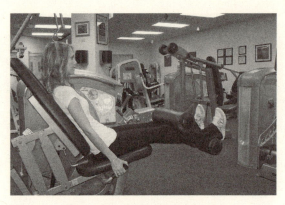

(Fig. 33)   Starting Position

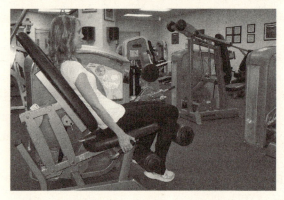

(Fig. 34)   Ending Position

More Choices for Your Workout

If neither free weights nor gym exercise equipment is the right form of exercise for you, go to my website where I have other suggestions for strength training that will melt the pounds away. Or if you would like to see some of the exercises on video, just download my Age-Defying Coach; it's free for my patients and readers (see page 294). Remember, my exercise programs will not bulk you up like a body-builder; they will make your body lean and firm while they turn back your metabolic clock.

CHAPTER 6

How Sleep Affects Your Metabolism and Your Weight

When new patients come to me for their first visit, they're surprised when I ask as many questions about their sleep patterns as I do about what they eat and how often they exercise. Getting a good night's sleep *every* night is now known to be crucial for psychological, cognitive, and metabolic health. Along with the right nutrition and proper exercise, sleep is the third pillar of wellness, and it's absolutely essential for rebooting your metabolism and losing that weight.

We've all met people or read about famous people who brag that they can get by with just a few hours of sleep every night. This type of sleep deprivation, known as short sleep, refers to getting fewer than six hours every night. Not getting enough regular sleep eventually catches up with these short sleepers as well as the rest of us.

Sleep deprivation is now the third leading cause of mortality, after smoking and after poor diet combined with a lack of exercise.

Adults who sleep five to seven hours per night or less are 30 to 80 percent more likely to develop Type 2 diabetes, cardiovascular disease, hypertension, and premature death as those who sleep eight hours or more. Chronic sleep deprivation increases appetite, blood pressure, and blood glucose levels, among other things. Those who don't sleep enough consume energy-rich foods, get a higher proportion of calories from fats or processed foods, and consume fewer fruits and vegetables, but more snacks. Study after study indicates that an unhealthy diet is associated with shorter sleep duration and irregular sleep patterns. When your sleep and your metabolism are disrupted, you can gain as much as 10 extra pounds per year.

With so many responsibilities—working, grocery shopping, cooking meals, helping with homework—there just isn't enough time during the day for us to accomplish everything. Not to mention all the hours we spend on our smartphones, tablets, and laptops. It's hard to unwind and rest well when you're checking electronic devices right before trying to get some shut-eye. Research shows checking email or social media right before bed contributes to poor sleep. Cutting back on sleep—as much as two to three hours a night—is the first thing people do to cram in all the other things they need to accomplish. (Of course, during times of stress or illness, your body and your brain need more sleep to heal.)

In addition to all the daily stress, hormonal changes that come as you get older make it seem nearly impossible to get a good night's sleep. You used to be asleep when your head hit the pillow, but now find that you're staring at the clock and counting sheep—yet you still can't get to sleep. You once slept through the night, but now you're roused several times by hormonal night sweats, a need to use the bathroom, or anxious thoughts racing through your mind. Poor sleep leaves you looking tired and feeling sluggish, makes you cranky, compromises your focus, slows your metabolism, and, yes, expands your waistline.

In this chapter, you'll discover the critical role that a good night's sleep plays in boosting your metabolism. You'll be introduced to simple habits as well as foods, beverages, and supplements that will help you get more restful sleep. You'll also learn which foods, beverages, and activities can disrupt your sleep cycle and should be avoided. In just three weeks, you'll be on your way to more restorative shut-eye, which can take years off your metabolic age. And you can achieve it without taking any medications.

Why Is Sleep Important?

Every spring, we get one hour less sleep as we shift to Daylight Saving Time. During the week after that shift, there is a 16 to 17 percent increase in motor vehicle accidents, some of them fatal. There is also a 5 percent increase in heart attacks that week. This phenomenon reverses come autumn when we gain one hour of sleep each night. Reported heart attacks drop by 5 percent. This is just one example of how sensitive the body and the brain are to sleep.

Babies and children, who need 12 hours of sleep for brain development and physical growth, are getting fewer hours every night, which affects learning and memory issues. With both parents working, children are often kept up well past their bedtimes so families can spend time together. Teenagers, who need nine hours of shut-eye, fall asleep at their school desks from lack of it, and then try to make up those lost hours with weekend sleep marathons. The Centers for Disease Control has called this mass insomnia a public health epidemic.

When we sleep, our brains are known to perform certain functions, such as memory building. Recent science shows that during sleep, the brain is cleaning out all of the clutter that accumulated during the day. We've all been told, "Don't make that phone call/ write that letter/send that email. Sleep on it and see how you feel in the morning." There's clearly more than a bit of truth in that piece of advice.

Each of us is born with an internal clock that regulates our circadian rhythm, the natural cycle of sleeping and waking hours. The production of the hormone melatonin, which is affected by light, helps our bodies differentiate night from day. Melatonin levels in our brains start to rise in the mid- to late evening, remain high for most of the night, and then decline in the early-morning hours as it becomes time to wake up. Production of melatonin levels gradually drops after the age of 30, contributing to sleep deprivation in your 30s, 40s, and beyond. But there are ways—manipulation of day and night, eating certain foods, avoiding certain foods, timing your meals, taking supplements, and reducing stress—to increase your body's melatonin production so you can get a solid night's sleep every night.

Other Hormones and Sleep

If you're a woman in the throes of midlife hormonal changes, you know how much harder it is to get a good night's sleep. Up to 40 percent of perimenopausal women and as many as 61 percent of post-menopausal women say they have trouble sleeping. While hot flashes and night sweats can be to blame, they aren't the only culprits. Depression, sleep apnea, restless leg syndrome, and a more frequent need to urinate in the middle of the night—all more common as you age—also contribute to sleepless nights.

It can be just as difficult for men to get some decent shut-eye. New evidence shows a link between dwindling testosterone levels in men over 50 and decreasing quality of sleep. According to a University of Montreal researcher, when you're a young man 10 to 20 percent of your total sleep is deep sleep. By the time you hit 50, deep sleep decreases to just 5 to 7 percent. And once you pass 60, you may not be getting any deep sleep at all. That not only leaves you feeling sluggish, mentally foggy, and grumpy, but also wreaks havoc with your metabolism.

When you aren't getting enough sleep, it can affect other hormones, too. Hunger hormones are primarily regulated while you sleep. Two hormones in particular, leptin and ghrelin, send appetite signals to your brain. Ghrelin levels rise to alert your brain that you're hungry. Leptin levels increase to send signals to your brain that you're satiated. Chronic lack of sleep has been shown to increase levels of ghrelin and cortisol and decrease levels of leptin and other satiety hormones.

When you skimp on sleep, it triggers the release of cortisol. Considered a stress hormone, cortisol stimulates the metabolism of carbohydrates and fats and is also involved in insulin production. All of these internal mechanisms can increase your appetite. If you routinely don't get enough sleep, cortisol levels can remain elevated, which translates into a bigger appetite and a bigger body.

Lack of Sleep Causes Metabolic Aging and Weight Gain

Sixty-year-old Mark came to see me about losing the 30 pounds that had settled around his middle over the last 10 years. He wanted to lose the weight for two reasons: Both of his parents died in their late 60s—his mother from heart disease, his father from the complications of Type 2 diabetes—and he was about to become a grandfather for the first time. Mark told me, "I want to be around to be able to play with the baby and any more grandchildren for a long time. Losing my parents when they were so young was devastating. They lost out on so much by not getting to watch their grandchildren grow up."

Mark had no problem sticking with the smoothies and whole-food meals. Like many men, he embraced my exercise routine and even added outdoor cycling to his schedule every other day. When Mark returned for his three-week checkup, he was dismayed to learn that he had lost only 10 pounds. "What's going on, Doc? I'm doing everything you told me to."

Not quite.

Mark had trouble falling asleep. As soon as he climbed into bed, all the worries—his business, customers he needed to get back to, money owed, money due him—popped into his head.

"It's so frustrating to toss and turn when I want to sleep. Everything starts to bother me once I turn out the lights. First, I think about work, then my mind wanders to my family. Then everything else—my wife's snoring, the light on the alarm clock, the traffic outside our window—keeps me from going to sleep. During the day I drink about six cups of coffee and a couple of cans of diet soda with caffeine to stay awake. I yawn during important meetings and have trouble staying focused. I fall asleep between 1 and 2 a.m., and then have to get up at 6 a.m."

One of the fastest ways to add years to your metabolic age and fat to your midsection is to skimp on how much sleep you get at night. Seven volunteers in a study that appeared in the *Annals of Internal Medicine* were asked to reduce the amount of time they slept from eight and a half hours to four and a half for four days. Reducing the number of hours they slept caused definitive changes in how their fat cells worked. When these people got less sleep, their fat cells became less sensitive to insulin, which is associated with an increased risk for obesity and Type 2 diabetes. In an article in the *New York Times*, the study's senior author Matthew Brady, an associate professor of medicine at the University of Chicago, said, "Metabolically, lack of sleep aged fat cells about 20 years."

The lack of sleep that causes metabolic aging also causes weight gain. If you routinely sleep fewer than five or six hours a night, you're more likely to have extra padding on your body. Newer findings show that you don't have to be chronically sleep-deprived to see and feel the effects. Just a few nights of bad sleep can cause the number on your scale to creep up almost instantly. How? Not getting enough sleep makes you feel hungrier and makes you consume more calories throughout the day. In a study in the *Proceedings of the National Academy of Sciences*, people who slept for only five hours ate 6 percent more calories than when they slept for nine hours.

Scientists are beginning to understand the biological and neurological mechanisms that cause you to gobble up a jumbo stack of chocolate chip pancakes drenched in syrup or grab a hunk of cheese after a restless night. Brain-imaging studies show that when you're sleep-deprived, your brain's reward centers respond differently to certain foods. The brain's reward centers play a critical role in human survival, driving you to engage in activities—such as eating, drinking, and having sex—that keep you alive and help propagate the species. Every time you do these things, your brain's reward centers release feel-good chemicals that encourage you to repeat the activity. When you aren't getting enough sleep, your reward centers respond more positively to foods like sweets and fatty fare than to a bowl of fruit. This becomes an endless cycle of eating unhealthy foods and getting positive feedback from the brain, which entices you to eat even more of those unhealthy foods.

Many studies also show that when you don't get the right amounts of deep sleep, areas of the brain involved in rational decision making become less active. This tends to make you more impulsive. So your reward centers make those sugary glazed doughnuts even more appealing to you than usual, and your rational brain is giving you the green light to eat as many as you want. That's a disastrous combination for your metabolic aging and weight.

Once Mark realized his sleep issues were getting in the way of rebooting his metabolism and losing weight, we worked out a get-more-sleep strategy. First, he stopped drinking beverages with caffeine by 2 p.m. for two days. Then he stopped by 1 p.m. for two days. Eventually, he allowed himself just one cup of coffee or one diet soda before 11 a.m. Two hours before bedtime, Mark made a list in a small notebook of all the things weighing on his mind and noted how he would handle the problem the next day. If there was a problem with a customer, Mark jotted down the client's email address or phone number with a sentence or two on what needed to be said. He turned his LED-faced alarm toward the wall and set the dimmer as low as possible. Mark also purchased a "pink noise" machine that emitted a soothing waterfall effect to calm his mind and body. Soft earplugs blocked the traffic noise as well as his wife's snoring. Pink noise is supposedly closer to sounds produced in nature like the ocean waves, as compared to white noise, which is a sound that contains every frequency within range of human hearing. Pink noise is more relaxing, whereas white noise is better at drowning out background sounds. Of course, Mark's sleep habits didn't change overnight, but by following the same routine every night for one month, he received the sleep necessary to reinvigorate his metabolism and lose weight. By eating the right foods, exercising, and making some lifestyle changes to achieve metabolically driven sleep, Mark lost the extra 20 pounds that were giving him such a hard time.

Snooze or Lose Your Metabolically
Active Lean Tissue

While you're sleeping at night, your body remains active, undergoing a number of important internal processes and preparing for the next day. Many of these processes are critical for repairing and developing lean muscle tissue, which has a major impact on your metabolism. As you slumber, your body pumps more blood into your muscles, which promotes their rebuilding and repair mechanisms. In addition, hormones are released that aid in the development of muscle tissue. All of these processes are vital to preserving the lean tissue that reboots your metabolism.

It's important to understand that every day of your life, your muscles are going through a never-ending cycle of breaking down the proteins within and regenerating new proteins to replace them. When you don't get enough shut-eye, your muscles don't receive the full benefit of the internal repair operations. Instead, your muscles can get stuck in breakdown mode.

New scientific evidence confirms that inadequate sleep leads to muscle loss, which slows metabolism and increases the chances that you will add fat to your middle section. The same *Annals of Internal Medicine* study mentioned earlier in this chapter that showed how insufficient sleep affects fat cells and insulin sensitivity also revealed a connection between a lack of sleep and muscle loss. The trial followed a group of overweight men and women in their 40s as they attempted to lose weight while maintaining lean muscle tissue. The researchers found that inadequate sleep impaired their efforts to burn fat without losing muscle. Compared with the group of volunteers who slept eight and a half hours a night, the group who slept only four and a half hours lost 60 percent more lean muscle tissue while losing 55 percent less fat. Getting adequate sleep is essential for maintaining metabolically active muscle tissue and losing more fat.

How Much Sleep Do You Need?

To get the maximum fat-burning and muscle-building effects of sleep, you need seven to eight hours of uninterrupted sleep every night.

For many people this means a big change in habits, and that's easier said than done. Before you head to the drugstore for over-the-counter or prescription sleep aids, try taking advantage of the foods, beverages, and everyday habits that act as natural sedatives and avoid the ones that energize you or disrupt your sleep cycle. Rest assured, if you follow this sleep prescription, a good night's rest awaits you.

What to Eat and Drink for a Good Night's Sleep

• **Protein:** Protein induces the releases of various gut hormones, such as CCK (cholecystokinin), ghrelin, and peptide tyrosine-tyrosine (PYY), which have been shown to have a significant effect on sleep. Scientists have found that the release of CCK after a high-fat, low-carbohydrate meal induced sleepiness. Ghrelin is best known as an appetite stimulator, but it is also involved in sleep-wake behavior. Research shows that PYY decreases wakefulness and enhances non-REM sleep. In one study, people who ate a low-protein diet for 48 hours took 21 minutes longer to reach the beneficial REM sleep stage. By eating protein as recommended on this program, your gut will release more of these hormones that are associated with improved sleep.

• **L-tryptophan:** This essential amino acid has been shown to help decrease the amount of time it takes to fall asleep, increase sleep time, and reduce the number of middle-of-the-night awakenings. Serotonin, a neurotransmitter that sends information to different parts of the brain, is known for its calming and drowsiness-inducing effects, and melatonin, a sleep-regulating hormone, can't be produced without L-tryptophan. Melatonin, in turn, requires carbohydrates and insulin to carry it to and through the blood-brain barrier to be effective. To help get a good night's sleep, eat foods that are rich in L-tryptophan, such as poultry, fish, red meat, eggs, and low-fat or nonfat cottage cheese and yogurt.

• **Tart cherry juice concentrate:** Antioxidant-rich tart cherries are one of the world's best sources of melatonin. Tart cherry juice concentrate, available in health food stores or online, has been shown to reduce insomnia and improve the quality and duration of sleep. Remember that it is a liquid *concentrate*; you must dilute it before you use it. Add 2 tablespoons to your evening smoothies, or dilute 2 tablespoons in 8 ounces of still or sparkling water and drink it at the end of your evening meal to help you get a better night's sleep.

• **Dairy:** Cow's milk, which contains melatonin, has long been considered a natural sedative. Its sleep-inducing qualities have been the subject of many studies. Some research shows benefits in terms of sleep duration and a reduced number of sleep interruptions when dairy is consumed prior to bedtime. On the Age-Defying Diet, stick with nonfat dairy products as potential sleep enhancers.

• **Whole grains:** Eating a small amount of whole grains at dinner may increase your brain's ability to absorb L-tryptophan. This may increase levels of sleep-promoting serotonin. Stick with the whole grains and the recommended serving size prescribed (½ cup cooked with whole-food meals).

• **Magnesium-rich foods:** Magnesium, a mineral known for its calming qualities, can help you switch off your busy mind so you can get to sleep. Many people don't get adequate amounts of magnesium as they age, because the ability to absorb it decreases and the body eliminates more of it when you urinate. Without enough of the quieting effects of magnesium, you may be more prone to sleepless nights. Approved magnesium-rich foods on this program include artichokes, brown rice, couscous, halibut, nonfat milk, oats, pearl barley, spinach, and whole wheat flour.

• **Herbal teas:** For centuries, people have been turning to herbal teas as relaxation and sleep aids. Many of my patients tell me that drinking a cup of chamomile or passionflower tea in the evening helps them relax, unwind, and fight off the temptation to snack.

Tips on How to Get a Good Night's Sleep

What to Do	Why
Make getting a good night's sleep a priority. Put it on your to-do list and cross it off just before turning off the lights.	Sleep is essential for rebooting your metabolism, as well as memory building and clearing out brain clutter every day.
Go to bed at the same time each night and get up at the same time each morning—weekends, too.	Frequent changes in your day-to-night routine promote insomnia.
Expose yourself to bright, natural sunlight or artificial light early in the morning. Minimize exposure to bright light at the end of the day.	Exposure to sunlight early in the day resets the body's internal clock each day. In the evening, minimizing exposure to light helps your internal body clock get ready for sleep.
Avoid strenuous physical exercise within two hours of going to bed. Some restorative yoga poses can be relaxing.	Strenuous exercise may stimulate catecholamines and other stress hormones and may interfere with sleep.
Make your bed irresistible, so you can't wait to climb into it. Purchase soft, comfortable bed linens and keep the bedroom quiet and cool (60 to 68°F).	The body's internal temperature drops to its lowest level during deep sleep. The sooner you can get to that stage, the more beneficial your night's sleep will be.

(continued)

What to Do	Why
Avoid caffeine within six to eight hours of bedtime.	It takes eight hours for coffee, tea, or soda with caffeine to be fully metabolized. Caffeine blocks the chemicals in your brain that promote sleep. To avoid caffeine-fueled sleeplessness, drink no more than one or two cups of coffee or other caffeinated beverages and have them before noon.
Avoid excess alcohol within six hours of sleep.	Although alcohol may initially facilitate sleep, it could disrupt sleep during the second half of the night.
If noise is a problem, get a pink noise machine or use a white noise smartphone app. Draw the shades or curtains or wear an eye mask. Reserve your bed for sleep and sex. Use low-wattage lightbulbs in the bedroom.	All of your senses need to be calm and quiet if you're to get a good night's sleep.
Have a small bedtime snack of foods high in tryptophan, like nonfat yogurt.	Foods high in tryptophan may help you sleep and help improve the quality of your sleep.
Create a relaxing bedtime ritual. Take a warm bath, learn to meditate, listen to classical music or quiet jazz, try some restorative yoga poses or guided imagery, or read a book by lamplight, not on a tablet or smartphone.	Knowing what to expect and following the same routine every night makes it easier to dismiss anxieties and fall asleep more easily.
Turn off the technology two hours before getting into bed.	Bright artificial light shining into your eyes from TVs, smartphones, tablets, computers, and gaming consoles makes your body think it's daytime and makes it harder to fall asleep.

What to Do	Why
If you have a lot of worries on your mind, write things down two hours before bedtime. If possible, include a short note on what you plan to do to resolve any problems.	Excessive stress and worries are associated with insomnia.
Avoid long naps. If you're tempted to take a nap, do some other activity instead of falling asleep in the middle of the day.	Napping for 10 to 20 minutes may be beneficial, but snoozing for an hour or more is apt to interfere with your ability to fall asleep or stay asleep through the night.
Sleep in as dark a room as possible.	Recent research has found that women had larger waistlines if their bedroom was "light enough to see across" at night.

Your Sleep
Follow the tips and eat the recommended foods above and try one of my Sleepytime SuperCharged Smoothies (pages 186–9) for your evening meal. (Eat your whole-food meal for breakfast or lunch, if it's not an all-smoothie day.)

Following these simple strategies should help you get more of the blissful sleep you need. If getting good sleep continues to be a problem, then you may have a sleep disorder, such as sleep apnea, insomnia, or RLS (restless leg syndrome). See a board-certified sleep medicine physician at a sleep center near you.

Sleep affects your hormone levels, your moods, and your weight. Getting enough and the right kind of shut-eye will help regulate your appetite hormones, reduce the levels of the fat-promoting hormone cortisol, increase muscle repair and regeneration, and lower your metabolic age.

Getting the proper amount of good sleep is important for losing weight. See the Age-Defying Coach (page 294) for more tips and even downloadable music so you get the sleep you need to help you lose weight.

CHAPTER 7

The Age-Defying Diet
Day by Day

Here are some menus that include the SuperCharged Smoothies, SuperCharged Soups, snacks, whole-food meals, and desserts that can be found in the recipe chapters of this book. Feel free to substitute a soup for a smoothie. You can also substitute tofu for chicken, or couscous for quinoa; there are many choices. You can always add an unlimited green or mixed vegetable salad or fruit to your whole-food meals. Remember, limit condiments to one serving. If you follow a vegan lifestyle, check out the plant-based protein powders suggested, starting on page 140. For more meal plans, custom menus, ready-made dessert options, and much more, visit my website DrApovian.com or download the Age-Defying Coach app. It is a free service for my patients, and I am happy that I can now also offer it free to you. (See page 294 to get your password.)

Your Snack

On all days other than your Supercharge Day, you may have a mid-afternoon snack of as much fruit and nonstarchy vegetables as you want (see pages 35–6). You may add one portion of a sauce or condiment (see page 280).

REBOOT: WEEK 1

DAY 1 Supercharger

Breakfast
Banana-Berry Bounty Smoothie (page 149)

Lunch
Pineapple Dream Smoothie (page 168) *or* Tomato-Herb Soup (page 207)

Dinner
Cherry-Almond Sleep Treat Smoothie (page 187) *or* Creamy Broccoli Soup (page 196)

DAY 2

Breakfast
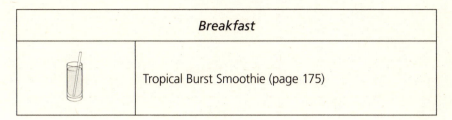 Tropical Burst Smoothie (page 175)

Lunch
Green Goodness Smoothie (page 161) *or* Courgette-Spinach Soup (page 208)

Snack
Citrus fruit salad *or* your choice of unlimited fruit and nonstarchy vegetables with one portion of a sauce or condiment (page 280)

Dinner
Garlic-Lemon Chicken (page 220) with roasted asparagus (page 246) and Whole Wheat Pasta (page 263) and one 6-ounce glass of wine *or* 12 ounces of beer *or* Raspberry Meringue Dessert (page 274) or a different ready-made dessert (page 264)

DAY 3

Breakfast
Blueberry-Pineapple-Choco-Coffee Blast (page 154)

Lunch
Living Green Smoothie (page 164) *or* Parsnip, Turnip, and Pear Soup (page 202)

Snack
Steamed mangetout with Tzatziki (page 288) *or* your choice of unlimited fruit and nonstarchy vegetables with one portion of a sauce or condiment (page 280)

Dinner
Turkey Meat Loaf (page 225) with Asian Slaw (page 242), cooked spring greens (page 248), and Quinoa (page 261) and one 6-ounce glass of wine *or* 12 ounces of beer *or* Pumpkin-Oat Cookies (page 273) or a different ready-made dessert (page 264)

DAY 4

Breakfast
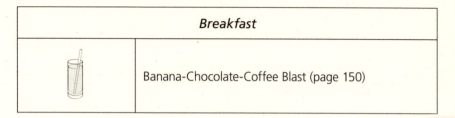 Banana-Chocolate-Coffee Blast (page 150)

Lunch
Spa Sipper Smoothie (page 170) *or* Tomato-Herb Soup (page 207)

Snack
Steamed broccoli florets (page 245) with Orange-Mint Yogurt Sauce (page 284) *or* your choice of unlimited fruit and nonstarchy vegetables with one portion of a sauce or condiment (page 280)

Dinner
Fish Fillets Baked in Foil Packets (page 230) with Couregette Noodles (page 255) and Amaranth (page 257) and one 6-ounce glass of wine *or* 12 ounces of beer *or* Strawberry Cheesecake Mousse (page 275) or a different ready-made dessert (page 264)

DAY 5

Breakfast	
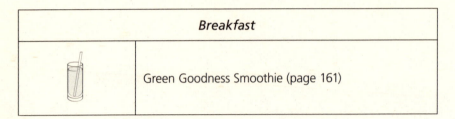	Green Goodness Smoothie (page 161)

Lunch	
or	Grape-Melon Mania Smoothie (page 158) *or* Asparagus Soup (page 191)

Snack	
	Apple Chips (page 277) *or* your choice of unlimited fruit and nonstarchy vegetables with one portion of a sauce or condiment (page 280)

Dinner	
plus or	Chicken with Red Grapes (page 218), Sautéed Spinach with Garlic (page 250), and Bulgur (page 259) and one 6-ounce glass of wine *or* 12 ounces of beer *or* No-Bake Kiwi Cookies (page 270) or a ready-made dessert (page 264)

DAY 6

Breakfast
Strawberry-Melon Magic Smoothie (page 172)

Lunch
Apple-Cucumber Refresher (page 148) *or* Roasted Red and Yellow Pepper Soup (page 203)

Snack
Papaya cubes with fresh lime juice and cracked pepper *or* your choice of unlimited fruit and nonstarchy vegetables with one portion of a sauce or condiment (page 280)

Dinner
Beef and Vegetable Kebabs (page 213), Quinoa (page 261), and mixed green salad and one 6-ounce glass of wine *or* 12 ounces of beer *or* Individual Peach Cobblers (page 267) or a different ready-made dessert (page 264)

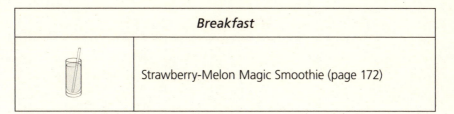

DAY 7

Breakfast
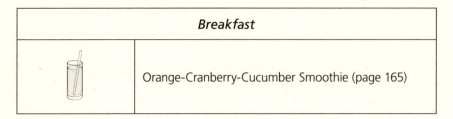 Orange-Cranberry-Cucumber Smoothie (page 165)

Lunch
or Green Tea–Berry Blend Smoothie (page 163) *or* Lentil, Tomato, and Spinach Soup (page 200)

Snack
Cherries dipped in nonfat plain yogurt *or* your choice of unlimited fruit and nonstarchy vegetables with one portion of a sauce or condiment (page 280)

Dinner
plus Chicken Breasts Stuffed with Ricotta Creamed Spinach (page 217), mixed green salad, and Whole Wheat Pasta (page 263) and one 6-ounce glass of wine *or* 12 ounces of beer *or* Cherry Fro-Yo (page 266) or a different ready-made dessert (page 264)

RECHARGE: WEEKS 2 AND 3

DAY 8 Supercharge

Breakfast
Tropical Burst Smoothie (page 175)

Lunch
Walking on Sunshine Smoothie (page 176) *or* Southwestern Soup (page 205)

Dinner
A Peachy Night's Sleep Smoothie (page 186) *or* Creamy Broccoli Soup (page 196)

DAY 9

Breakfast

	Meet Your Matcha Smoothie (page 184)

Lunch

	Waldorf Chicken Salad (page 244) on a bed of baby greens

Snack

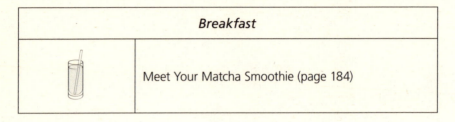	Steamed green beans (page 245) with Pesto (page 286) or your choice of unlimited fruit and nonstarchy vegetables with one portion of a sauce or condiment (page 280)

Dinner

| plus

or | Chicken Breasts Baked in Foil Packets (page 215), Cooked Greens (page 248), and Quinoa (page 261) with Tomato Sauce (page 287) and

one 6-ounce glass of wine or

12 ounces of beer or

Chocolate Crisps (page 286) or a different ready-made dessert (page 264) |
|---|---|

DAY 10

Breakfast
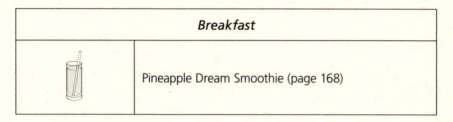 Pineapple Dream Smoothie (page 168)

Lunch
or A Glass of Health Smoothie (page 147) Cauliflower and Roasted Garlic Soup (page 195)

Snack
Grapefruit segments with Orange-Mint Yogurt Sauce (page 284) *or* your choice of unlimited fruit and nonstarchy vegetables with one portion of a sauce or condiment (page 280)

Dinner
plus or Grilled salmon, spinach salad with red onions, Dijon Mustard Lemon Dressing (page 281), and Tabbouleh (page 262) and one 6-ounce glass of wine *or* 12 ounces of beer *or* Pecan-Flax Crookers (page 269) or a different ready-made dessert (page 264)

DAY 11

Breakfast
Winter Fresh Smoothie (page 177)

Lunch
Rocket, watercress, and radicchio with grilled shrimp and Dijon Mustard Lemon Dressing (page 281) and steamed green beans (page 245)

Snack
Endive leaves with Roasted Aubergine (page 253) *or* your choice of unlimited fruit and nonstarchy vegetables with one portion of a sauce or condiment (page 280)

Dinner
Oven-Roasted Tofu on Baby Spinach (page 239) and Brown Rice (page 258) and
one 6-ounce glass of wine *or*
12 ounces of beer *or*
Peanut-Butter-and-Chocolate-Drizzled Bananas (page 271) or a different ready-made dessert (page 264)

plus

or

DAY 12

Breakfast
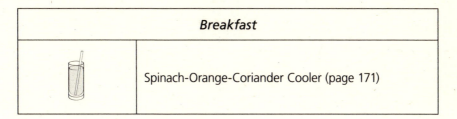 Spinach-Orange-Coriander Cooler (page 171)

Lunch
Spa Sipper Smoothie (page 170) *or*   Carrot, Peach, and Ginger Soup (page 193)

Snack
Cucumber slices with Tzatziki (page 288) *or* your choice of unlimited fruit and nonstarchy vegetables with one portion of a sauce or condiment (page 280)

Dinner
Turkey Meat Loaf (page 225), Sautéed Spinach with Garlic (page 250), roast carrots (page 246), and Couscous (page 260) and   one 6-ounce glass of wine *or*   12 ounces of beer *or*   Pineapple-Coconut Cupcakes (page 276) or a different ready-made dessert (page 264)

DAY 13

Breakfast
Raspberry-Orange Refresher (page 169)

Lunch
Leftover Turkey Meat Loaf (page 225) with Steamed Baby Pak Choi (page 252) and Brown Rice (page 258)

Snack
Fennel leaves with Dijon Mustard Lemon Dressing (page 281) *or* your choice of unlimited fruit and nonstarchy vegetables with one portion of a sauce or condiment (page 280)

Dinner
Roasted Pork Tenderloin (page 226), roasted cauliflower (page 246), Coleslaw (page 243), and Quinoa (page 261) and
one 6-ounce glass of wine *or*
12 ounces of beer *or*
Melon Ribbons (page 278) or a different ready-made dessert (page 264)

plus

or

DAY 14

Breakfast

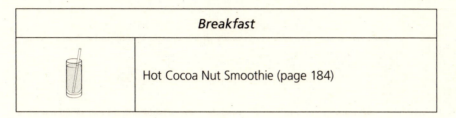	Hot Cocoa Nut Smoothie (page 184)

Lunch

	Banana-Berry Bounty Smoothie (page 149) *or*
or	Broccoli-Spinach Soup (page 192)

Snack

	Broccoli with Lemon-Artichoke Sauce (page 283) *or* your choice of unlimited fruit and nonstarchy vegetables with one portion of a sauce or condiment (page 280)

Dinner

	Roasted Turkey Breast (page 222) with Mango Salsa (page 289), cooked kale (page 248), and Brown Rice (page 258) and
plus	one 6-ounce glass of wine *or*
	12 ounces of beer *or*
or	Roasted Peaches (page 279) or a different ready-made dessert (page 264)

DAY 15 Supercharge

Breakfast	
	Grapes 'n' Greens Smoothie (page 159)

Lunch	
or	Cucumber-Melon-Mango Cooler (page 156) *or* Asparagus Soup (page 191)

Dinner	
or	Berry Fine Shake (page 153) *or* Southwestern Soup (page 205)

DAY 16

Breakfast

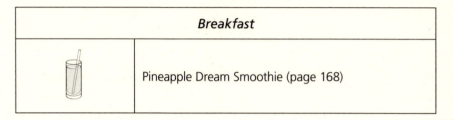

Pineapple Dream Smoothie (page 168)

Lunch

Green salad topped with leftover Roasted Turkey Breast (page 222), cucumbers, tomatoes, and steamed green beans with Dijon Mustard Lemon Dressing (page 281)

Snack

Jicama (or turnip) and carrot sticks with Pico de Gallo (page 290) *or* your choice of unlimited fruit and nonstarchy vegetables with one portion of a sauce or condiment (page 280)

Dinner

Boiled Shrimp (page 233), Asian Slaw (page 242), Steamed Baby Pak Choi (page 252), and Brown Rice (page 258) and

plus

one 6-ounce glass of wine *or*

12 ounces of beer *or*

or

Pear-Chai Pudding (page 272) or a different ready-made dessert (page 264)

DAY 17

Breakfast

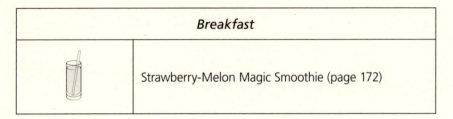	Strawberry-Melon Magic Smoothie (page 172)

Lunch

	Berry-Banana Freeze Smoothie (page 152) *or*
or	Creamy Mushroom Soup (page 197)

Snack

	Cantaloupe cubes with Orange-Mint Yogurt Sauce (page 284) *or* your choice of unlimited fruit and nonstarchy vegetables with one portion of a sauce or condiment (page 280)

Dinner

	Grilled tuna with Mango Salsa (page 289), grilled vegetables, and Amaranth (page 257) and
plus	one 6-ounce glass of wine *or*
	12 ounces of beer *or*
or	Pecan-Flax Crookers (page 269) or a different ready-made dessert (page 264)

DAY 18

Breakfast
Cherry-Banana Blast (page 155)

Lunch
Waldorf Chicken Salad (page 244) on rocket, radicchio, and endive

Snack
Grapes dipped in nonfat yogurt *or* your choice of unlimited fruit and nonstarchy vegetables with one portion of a sauce or condiment (page 280)

Dinner
Baked Whole Fish (page 232) with Pico de Gallo (page 290), Roasted Vegetables (page 246), cucumber and tomato salad, and Quinoa (page 261) and
one 6-ounce glass of wine *or*
12 ounces of beer *or*
Blueberry Pie Cups (page 265) or a different ready-made dessert (page 264)

plus

or

DAY 19

Breakfast
Winter Fresh Smoothie (page 177)

Lunch
Strawberry-Peach-Cucumber Cooler (page 173) *or*   Carrot, Pumpkin, and Apple Soup (page 194)

Snack
Cherry tomatoes drizzled with Pesto (page 286) *or* your choice of unlimited fruit and nonstarchy vegetables with one portion of a sauce or condiment (page 280)

Dinner
Sirloin Steaks with Mushroom Sauce (page 211), roasted broccoli and cauliflower (page 246) and Brown Rice (page 258) and
one 6-ounce glass of wine *or*
12 ounces of beer *or*
Cherry Fro-Yo (page 266) or a different ready-made dessert (page 264)

DAY 20

Breakfast

	Banana-Berry Bounty Smoothie (page 149)

Lunch

	1 can tuna mixed with Mayonnaise (page 282) and chopped spring onions, celery, and parsley and served on a bed of baby greens with radishes and tomatoes

Snack

	Grilled pineapple rings *or* your choice of unlimited fruit and nonstarchy vegetables with one portion of a sauce or condiment (page 280)

Dinner

	Pork Chops with Dijon Mustard Sauce (page 228), roasted mushrooms and onions (page 246), steamed mangetout peas (page 245), and
plus	one 6-ounce glass of wine *or*
	12 ounces of beer *or*
or	Roasted Peaches (page 279) or a different ready-made dessert (page 264)

DAY 21

Breakfast	
	Strawberry Sipper (page 174)

Lunch	
or	Green Goodness Smoothie (page 161) *or* Kale, Spinach, and Tomato Soup (page 199)

Snack	
	Steamed broccoli florets (page 245) with Lemon-Artichoke Sauce (page 283) *or* your choice of unlimited fruit and nonstarchy vegetables with one portion of a sauce or condiment (page 280)

Dinner	
plus or	Grilled salmon fillet and spring onions, roasted brussels sprouts and carrots (page 246), and Quinoa (page 261) and one 6-ounce glass of wine *or* 12 ounces of beer *or* Raspberry Meringue Dessert (page 274) or a different ready-made dessert (page 264)

REVITALIZE: STAYING YOUNGER AND THINNER FOR LIFE

DAY 22 Supercharge

	Breakfast
	Banana-Chocolate-Coffee Blast (page 150)

	Lunch
or	Green Apple Reboot Smoothie (page 160) *or* Tomato-Herb Soup (page 207)

	Dinner
or	Citrus Sleeper Smoothie (page 189) *or* Curried Courgette-Cauliflower Soup (page 198)

DAY 23

Breakfast	
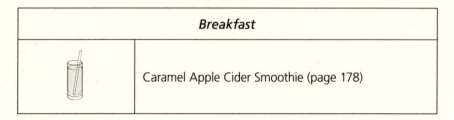	Caramel Apple Cider Smoothie (page 178)

Lunch	
	Mixed green salad topped with sliced Sirloin Steak (page 211), tomatoes, cucumbers, and red onion

Snack	
	Diced apple, celery, and grape salad with Mayonnaise (page 285) *or* your choice of unlimited fruit and nonstarchy vegetables with one portion of a sauce or condiment (page 282)

Dinner	
plus or	Spicy Lemon Trout Fillets (page 231), Sautéed Spinach with Garlic (page 250), and Tabbouleh (page 262) and one 6-ounce glass of wine *or* 12 ounces of beer *or* Pumpkin-Oat Cookies (page 273) or a different ready-made dessert (page 264)

DAY 24

Breakfast
Creamy Chai Smoothie (page 181)

Lunch
Open-Faced Turkey-Portobello Burger (page 223) with lettuce, tomatoes, cucumbers, and pickles

Snack
Mixed fruit salad *or* your choice of unlimited fruit and nonstarchy vegetables with one portion of a sauce or condiment (page 280)

Dinner
Boiled Shrimp (page 233), Swiss chard, and Brown Rice (page 258) and
one 6-ounce glass of wine *or*
12 ounces of beer *or*
Pear-Chai Pudding (page 272) or a different ready-made dessert (page 264)

plus

or

DAY 25

Breakfast
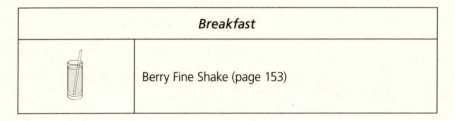 Berry Fine Shake (page 153)

Lunch
Bowl of tossed salad with leftover Boiled Shrimp (page 233)

Snack
Steamed cauliflower and broccoli (page 245) with Mayonnaise (page 282) *or* your choice of unlimited fruit and nonstarchy vegetables with one portion of a sauce or condiment (page 280)

Dinner
Sirloin Steaks with Mushroom Sauce (page 211), Sautéed Spinach with Garlic (page 250), and mixed green salad, and
plus
one 6-ounce glass of wine *or*
12 ounces of beer *or*
Strawberry Cheesecake Mousse (page 275) or a different ready-made dessert (page 264)

DAY 26

Breakfast
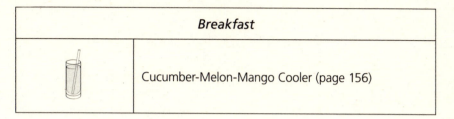 Cucumber-Melon-Mango Cooler (page 156)

Lunch
1 can tuna, packed in water, drained, and mixed with Mayonnaise (page 282) and celery on cos lettuce leaves with cherry tomatoes and sliced cucumbers

Snack
Pepper wedges and cucumbers with Pico de Gallo (page 290) *or* your choice of unlimited fruit or nonstarchy vegetables and one portion of a sauce or condiment (page 280)

Dinner
Chicken Breasts Baked in Foil Packets (page 215) with green beans and summer squash and Quinoa (page 261) and
plus
one 6-ounce glass of wine *or*
12 ounces of beer *or*
or
Peanut-Butter-and-Chocolate-Drizzled Bananas (page 271) or a different ready-made dessert (page 264)

DAY 27

Breakfast
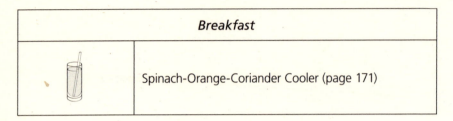 Spinach-Orange-Coriander Cooler (page 171)

Lunch
Waldorf Chicken or Turkey Salad (page 244) on a bed of baby spinach

Snack
Mixed berries with Orange-Mint Yogurt Sauce (page 284) *or* your choice of unlimited fruit and vegetables with one portion of a sauce or condiment (page 280)

Dinner
Roasted Pork Tenderloin (page 226) with Mango Salsa (page 289), roasted carrots and cauliflower (page 246), Coleslaw (page 243), and Quinoa (page 261) and
one 6-ounce glass of wine *or*
12 ounces of beer *or*
No-Bake Kiwi Cookies (page 270) or a different ready-made dessert (page 264)

plus

or

DAY 28

Breakfast
Orange Juiced-Up Smoothie (page 166)

Lunch
Roasted Turkey Breast (page 222), Quinoa (page 261), lettuce, and tomatoes

Snack
Apple, kiwi, and strawberry fruit salad *or* your choice of unlimited fruit and nonstarchy vegetables with one portion of a sauce or condiment (page 280)

Dinner
Halibut Fillets Baked in Foil Packets (page 230) and Brown Rice (page 258) and
one 6-ounce glass of wine *or*
12 ounces of beer *or*
No-Bake Kiwi Cookies (page 270) or a different ready-made dessert (page 264)

plus

or

Find alternative meal plans at DrApovian.com.

CHAPTER 8

SuperCharged Smoothies

When I tell new patients that they'll be drinking smoothies—lots of delicious, filling smoothies—to lose weight with the Age-Defying Diet, they don't believe me. But once they start making, shaking, and drinking my protein-packed, fiber-rich SuperCharged Smoothies, they're amazed at the great taste and how quickly they shed weight.

These easy-to-make SuperCharged Smoothies are the key to losing weight successfully, quickly, and safely. Because they're packed with nutritious fruits and vegetables, vital nutrients, and essential ingredients that fight hunger and cravings, these flavorful meal replacements give you all the benefits of intermittent fasting but without the sacrifice of skipping meals. Age-Defying Diet smoothies couldn't be easier. You just combine the ingredients in a blender and voilà—you've got a satisfying meal that will help you lose pounds and inches.

A Top-Quality Protein Powder Is Essential

Walk into any health or vitamin store, and the number of protein powders to choose from can be overwhelming. Some are made from animal-source proteins, while vegetarian versions are made from soya, peas, rice, or hemp. Some proteins contain artificial flavorings and sweeteners, while others have few additives. The protein powder you put into your smoothies is a key component to your weight loss success.

Types of Protein Powders and Recommended Brands

Below I describe the different protein powders available. You can choose any reliable brand and be successful on the Age-Defying Diet. Be sure to use only unflavored protein powders with no sugar added. A blend is your best choice.

Whey and Casein Blend

I recommend whey and casein blend as the best protein for your shakes. Whey and casein have different but complementary effects. Whey is a fast-digesting, complete protein that provides all the amino acids your body needs. It has particularly high levels of the amino acid leucine, which stimulates the protein synthesis that helps protect lean muscle tissue and re-ignite metabolism. Casein is another complete protein, offering a full range of amino acids, including a particularly healthy dose of glutamine. One of the greatest benefits of casein is that it is slowly digested, which means it can provide a steady flow of amino acids to your muscles for hours. In addition to maintaining muscle mass—key to rebooting your metabolism—casein's slow-release action helps keep hunger at bay and enhances fat loss. When you combine the two, you receive the benefits of both to speed up your metabolism. You can mix your own by combining two good unflavored whey or caesin products. Just mix 50 percent of one serving of unflavored whey protein powder and 50 percent of one serving of unflavored casein protein powder. The total should contain no less than 20 grams of protein. You can also try adding these booster ingredients to your smoothie mixes.

- **Flaxseed:** Rich in omega-3 fatty acids, flaxseed helps fuel weight loss. Mountains of scientific evidence suggest that consuming omega-3 fatty acids, found in flaxseeds, improves the body's ability to burn fat and drop pounds. Omega-3s also play a role in satiety, keeping you feeling fuller longer. Flaxseed is the richest source of the plant-based omega-3 fatty acid alpha-linoleic acid (ALA).

- **Vitamins and minerals:** Essential vitamins and minerals—vitamins A, B_6, B_{12}, C, D, E, and K; and calcium, folate, potassium, magnesium, manganese, thiamin, and zinc—promote good health, boost immunity, and supercharge energy.

- **Glucomannan (konjac flour):** It's a natural thickening agent. This "secret" ingredient has been called one of nature's best appetite suppressants. Glucomannan is a sugar derived from the konjac plant (also called yam cake). When digested, it acts like a sponge and absorbs water to form a bulky fiber. This sponginess reduces the absorption of carbohydrates and cholesterol. Glucomannan has also been shown to lower cholesterol, help balance blood sugar in Type 2 diabetes, and relieve constipation.

Use this mix as a base for the recipes, or use a reliable brand of protein powder.

Plant-Based Protein Powders

If you're a vegetarian, vegan, or prefer not to use an animal-product-based protein powder, there are many plant-based options available.

Soya protein powder: Known for their antioxidant powers, soya protein powders contain all of the essential and nonessential amino acids that make up a complete protein. Many soya protein powders, however, contain less than the 20 grams of protein per serving that I find necessary to boost your metabolism and burn fat. Always check the nutrition label of soya protein powder to see how many grams of protein are provided in one serving. Note that soya protein powder is not recommended for men on this program. Studies have shown that excessive intake of soya products can cause hormonal changes in men, increasing their estrogen levels beyond those of a healthy female.

50/50 blend of pea and brown rice protein powders: This blended protein powder mix provides a nutritionally complete, plant-based protein powder that contains all essential amino acids to provide optimum muscle protection and boost your metabolism. Individually, pea protein powder and brown rice protein powder are considered incomplete proteins that will not spur the permanent, fast-acting weight loss you will experience on this program. Together, they work powerfully.

Hemp: It's a plant-based protein powder that contains all the essential amino acids your body needs. This superfood is rich in omega-3 fatty acids and fiber, as well as iron and calcium. Be sure to look for unhulled hemp seed powder, which is considered more digestible than other hemp seed proteins.

Egg protein: Available as a powder, it contains all essential amino acids and is a complete source of protein. Since it has no whey or casein, egg protein is naturally free of lactose, making it easier to digest for those who are lactose-intolerant. On the other hand, some people have egg-related allergies and sensitivities including gas, bloating, and other gastrointestinal distress, making egg protein unsuitable for them.

Nonfat Greek yogurt: To add more variety to your smoothies, you can use plain, nonfat Greek yogurt. Creamy, tasty, and packed with about 15 to 20 grams of protein per 6-ounce serving, this can be used as a source of protein in your smoothies. Greek yogurt is also known for its probiotics, biologically active cultures that aid in digestion and support the immune system.

Protein Powder

At least 20 grams of protein per serving. Only use unflavored protein powder containing no more than 120 calories with no added sugar.

Other Smoothie Ingredients

Once you determine which protein powder is right for you, here's a handy list of the other ingredients you'll need to make smoothies.

Liquid Action

When it comes to adding liquids to your smoothies, you have many options. They include water, unsweetened coconut water, fat-free or low-fat milk, and fat-free or low-fat dairy unsweetened alternatives— such as soya milk, unsweetened almond milk, or coconut milk. You can also add ice for a truly refreshing warm-weather smoothie.

Fruits and Vegetables

Fruits and vegetables are filled with hunger-fighting fiber and jam-packed with health-promoting vitamins and antioxidants yet are low in calories and fat.

Fresh fruits and vegetables: Whether from your own garden, your local farmers' market, or your grocery store, fresh produce is ideal for your smoothies. Wash all produce thoroughly. If you're using organic produce, retain the edible skins. The pulp and skins contain all the good-for-you fiber, which is part of what helps keep you feeling full for hours, keeps your digestive system moving, and promotes good health. This is the reason that juices are not included on the Age-Defying Diet. Use produce within a reasonable amount of time for best results.

Frozen fruits and vegetables: Keep bags of frozen berries, mangoes, pineapples, and other fruits in your freezer. When buying frozen foods, check the nutrition labels to make sure they contain no added sugar or fat. One of my favorite tips is to peel and freeze overripe bananas. A frozen banana adds a slightly sweet flavor and a creamy texture.

Canned fruits and vegetables: Checking nutrition labels is a must when you're using canned goods—they are often packed in syrup and high in sodium. Consuming too much sodium can lead to water retention and bloating, which is counterproductive to your efforts to lose that belly fat. Opt for foods that are water-packed, or packed in their own juices. Not in syrup and no added sugar; low-sodium brands only.

An Extra Drop of Flavor

Love the taste of cinnamon? Crave the tropical flavor of coconut? Dream about almond butter? You can season your smoothies with ¼ to ½ teaspoon of ground spices, such as cardamom, cinnamon, ginger, nutmeg, or a dash of unsweetened flavoring extract, such as almond, amaretto, cherry, coconut, lemon, orange, maple, or vanilla.

A Hint of Sweetness

If you like your smoothies on the sweeter side, add a bit of no-calorie sweetener, such as stevia or Splenda, when blending your beverages. Stevia, which comes from the plant of the same name, is very sweet, so a little bit goes a long way.

Choosing a Blender

Because smoothies are so important to your success on the Age-Defying Diet program, invest in a durable blender with a solid, heavy blade that has enough power to puree solid carrots, fibrous celery, and frozen fruits, as well as crushing ice. Blenders range in price from £20 to hundreds of pounds. Also consider a smaller, portable blender or shaker to keep in your desk or your car, so you can whip up a smoothie at your convenience. For more information on which blender is right for you, visit my website DrApovian.com.

Perfect Age-Defying Diet Smoothies

Want to know the secrets of making a well-blended smoothie? Put the ingredients into the blender in the order directed, and say good-bye to those lumps of fruit and clumps of protein powder. Here's how:

1. **Liquids.** Whether you're using fat-free milk, unsweetened coconut water, unsweetened almond milk, or water, put the liquid in the blender first.
2. **Fruits and vegetables.** Add the heaviest fruits and vegetables first, followed by the lightest. For example, if you're making a smoothie with frozen bananas, fresh strawberries, and a handful of fresh spinach leaves, start with the frozen bananas because they're the densest, followed by the strawberries, and then the spinach leaves.

3. **Protein powder.** Add your protein powder now.
4. **Flavorings.** Ground spices or extracts.
5. **Ice or water.** If you like thick smoothies, add three or four ice cubes when you're almost done blending. If the smoothie is too thick once it's blended, thin it out with a few tablespoons of water.

If you're using a blend-and-go blender, you may need to add bulkier ingredients little by little to avoid clogging up the machine and to ensure smooth blending.

Other Smoothie Tips

• Save money by purchasing frozen fruits—such as mango cubes and berries—and vegetables like kale and spinach in large, economical bags at big-box stores, where they're available year-round.

• Double the smoothie recipe and freeze each portion in individual containers or freezer bags. Place a frozen smoothie in the refrigerator overnight to thaw. It will be ready to drink by morning. Give the thawed smoothie a few good shakes, as some ingredients may have separated over time. Drink frozen smoothies within seven days.

• Wash all fruits and vegetables well before using. Dark leafy greens, such as kale, spinach, and rocket, are grown in sandy soil and need to be thoroughly cleaned. For kale and spinach, remove and discard the tough stems from the greens. Fill a salad spinner with cool water and add the greens, pressing down to submerge them. Lift out the basket. Rinse out the salad spinner bowl well. Repeat with fresh water until no dirt is left on the bottom of the spinner.

• If you prefer, you can use frozen, instead of fresh, spinach or kale as well as frozen fruits such as mangoes, pineapples, berries, melons, kiwis, peaches, and so on. Frozen fruits and vegetables will give your smoothies a rich, creamy texture, making it unnecessary to use ice cubes.

• When bananas, mangoes, and other fruits become overripe, don't toss them out! Peel and freeze them in plastic bags for your smoothies. If you're freezing a larger fruit like a mango or a pear, be sure to peel (if necessary) and cut the fruit before freezing.

• Whether fresh, frozen, or canned, pieces of fruits and vegetables should be cut into sizes recommended by the manufacturer of your blender. Obviously, a blender with a high-powered, high-performance motor can handle larger pieces than a model with a smaller motor. Bananas and carrots should be peeled and cut into chunks before they are added to the blender. Apples and pears should be cut up and seeded—but leave the skins on since that's where a lot of the fruits' nutrition is. Citrus fruits such as oranges, grapefruits, and tangerines should be peeled, segmented, and depipped.

• From fruit smoothies bursting with fresh fruit flavor and nutrition to green smoothies chock-full of their own vital nutrients, my protein smoothie recipes will keep your metabolism humming and the weight melting off, all while tasting delicious and leaving you feeling full and content. Every smoothie in this chapter can be enjoyed for breakfast, lunch, or dinner. Each one is formulated to pack the maximum amount of protein, nutrition, and flavor into every glass no matter what recipes you choose.

SUPERCHARGED SMOOTHIE RECIPES

(see page 297 for measurement conversions)

A Glass of Health Smoothie

½ cup water

1 cup fresh orange juice

1 serving smoothie mix (pages 139–40) or 1 serving other protein
 powder

1 cup chopped cos lettuce leaves

½ cup fresh or frozen blueberries

1 cup fresh or frozen strawberries

1 carrot, chopped

Put all the ingredients in the blender in the order they are listed. Process on high speed until the mixture is smooth, adding water and/or ice as needed to achieve the desired consistency.

Protein: 24g • Calories: 345 • Dietary Fiber: 13g

Apple-Cucumber Refresher

½ cup brewed and cooled unsweetened green tea or water

1 serving smoothie mix (pages 139–40) or 1 serving other protein powder

1 cup chopped cos lettuce leaves

1 cup cucumber chunks

2½ apples, cored and chopped

Put all the ingredients in the blender in the order they are listed. Process on high speed until the mixture is smooth, adding water and/or ice as needed to achieve the desired consistency.

Protein: 22g • Calories: 321 • Dietary Fiber: 11g

Banana-Berry Bounty Smoothie

½ cup water

1 serving smoothie mix (pages 139–40) or 1 serving other protein powder

2 cups packed baby spinach or frozen chopped spinach

1¼ cups fresh or frozen blueberries

1¼ bananas, peeled

Put all the ingredients in the blender in the order they are listed. Process on high speed until the mixture is smooth, adding water and/or ice as needed to achieve the desired consistency.

Protein: 25g • Calories: 361 • Dietary Fiber: 15g

Banana-Chocolate-Coffee Blast

1 cup unsweetened almond milk

½ cup water

1½ teaspoons vanilla extract

1 serving smoothie mix (pages 139–40) or 1 serving other protein
  powder

2 tablespoons unsweetened cocoa powder

2 teaspoons espresso powder or 2 tablespoons brewed strong
  black coffee, cooled

1 banana, peeled

½ cup fresh or frozen sliced peaches

¼ cup peeled, roughly chopped fresh or frozen carrots

½ cup frozen chopped mustard greens

Put all the ingredients in the blender in the order they are listed. Process on high speed until the mixture is smooth, adding water and/or ice as needed to achieve the desired consistency.

Protein: 26g • Calories: 347 • Dietary Fiber: 16g

Banana-Strawberry-Ginger Blast

½ cup water

1 serving smoothie mix (pages 139–40) or 1 serving other protein
  powder

2¼ teaspoons chopped fresh ginger

1½ bananas, peeled

1½ cups fresh or frozen strawberries

1½ cups baby spinach or frozen chopped spinach

Put all the ingredients in the blender in the order they are listed. Process on high speed until the mixture is smooth, adding water and/or ice as needed to achieve the desired consistency.

Protein: 25g • Calories: 354 • Dietary Fiber: 15g

Berry-Banana Freeze Smoothie

½ cup water

1 serving smoothie mix (pages 139–40) or 1 serving other protein powder

1 teaspoon fresh lemon juice

2 cups fresh or frozen kale leaves

1 cup fresh or frozen strawberries

1 banana, peeled

Put all the ingredients in the blender in the order they are listed. Process on high speed until the mixture is smooth, adding water and/or ice as needed to achieve the desired consistency.

Protein: 27g • Calories: 332 • Dietary Fiber: 14g

Berry Fine Shake

½ cup water

2 tablespoons lemon juice

1 serving smoothie mix (pages 139–40) or 1 serving other protein
   powder

2 cups fresh or frozen spinach

1½ cups fresh or frozen blueberries

1½ cups fresh or frozen strawberries

Put all the ingredients in the blender in the order they are listed. Process on high speed until the mixture is smooth, adding water and/or ice as needed to achieve the desired consistency.

Protein: 25g • Calories: 330 • Dietary Fiber: 16g

Blueberry-Pineapple-Choco-Coffee Blast

½ cup water

1 serving smoothie mix (pages 139–40) or 1 serving other protein powder

¼ cup canned pumpkin puree (not pumpkin pie filling)

1 teaspoon pure vanilla extract

2 tablespoons unsweetened cocoa powder

2 teaspoons espresso powder or 2 tablespoons brewed strong black coffee, cooled

1 cup fresh or frozen blueberries

¾ cup fresh or frozen pineapple, or canned unsweetened pineapple slices, drained

1 cup frozen chopped fresh or frozen kale or mustard greens

Put all the ingredients in the blender in the order they are listed. Process on high speed until the mixture is smooth, adding water and/or ice as needed to achieve the desired consistency.

Protein: 26g • Calories: 333 • Dietary Fiber: 15g

Cherry-Banana Blast

½ cup water

1 serving smoothie mix (pages 139–40) or 1 serving other protein powder

2 cups fresh or frozen spinach

1¼ cups pitted cherries

1 banana, peeled

Put all the ingredients in the blender in the order they are listed. Process on high speed until the mixture is smooth, adding water and/or ice as needed to achieve the desired consistency.

Protein: 25g • Calories: 350 • Dietary Fiber: 13g

Cucumber-Melon-Mango Cooler

½ cup water

1 serving smoothie mix (pages 139–40) or 1 serving other protein
  powder

1 tablespoon fresh lemon juice

1 cup fresh or frozen spinach

1 cup cucumber chunks

1½ cups fresh or frozen mango cubes

1 cup melon cubes

Put all the ingredients in the blender in the order they are listed. Process on high speed until the mixture is smooth, adding water and/or ice as needed to achieve the desired consistency.

Protein: 24g • Calories: 351 • Dietary Fiber: 13g

Fruity Green Tea Smoothie

1 cup brewed and cooled unsweetened green tea

1 serving smoothie mix (pages 139–40) or 1 serving other protein powder

1 cup fresh or frozen spinach

1 cup fresh or frozen mango cubes

1 banana, peeled

Put all the ingredients in the blender in the order they are listed. Process on high speed until the mixture is smooth, adding water and/or ice as needed to achieve the desired consistency.

Protein: 23g • Calories: 332 • Dietary Fiber: 12g

Grape-Melon Mania Smoothie

½ cup water

1 serving smoothie mix (pages 139–40) or 1 serving other protein
    powder

2 cups chopped cos lettuce leaves

1½ cups seedless grapes

1 cup cantaloupe cubes

Put all the ingredients in the blender in the order they are listed. Process on high speed until the mixture is smooth, adding water and/or ice as needed to achieve the desired consistency.

Protein: 24g • Calories: 337 • Dietary Fiber: 10g

Grapes 'n' Greens Smoothie

½ cup water

1 serving smoothie mix (pages 139–40) or 1 serving other protein powder

1 teaspoon fresh lime juice

1 cup chopped cos lettuce leaves

1 cup cucumber chunks

1 apple, halved and cored

1¼ cups seedless grapes

Put all the ingredients in the blender in the order they are listed. Process on high speed until the mixture is smooth, adding water and/or ice as needed to achieve the desired consistency.

Protein: 23g • Calories: 343 • Dietary Fiber: 11g

Green Apple Reboot Smoothie

½ cup water

1 serving smoothie mix (pages 139–40) or 1 serving other protein
    powder

½ cup chopped cos lettuce leaves

1½ cups cucumber chunks

1½ cups fresh or frozen pineapple cubes

1 apple, halved and cored

Put all the ingredients in the blender in the order they are listed. Process on high speed until the mixture is smooth, adding water and/or ice as needed to achieve the desired consistency.

Protein: 23g • Calories: 339 • Dietary Fiber: 12g

Green Goodness Smoothie

½ cup unsweetened coconut water

½ cup water

1 serving smoothie mix (pages 139–40) or 1 serving other protein
  powder

1 cup chopped cos lettuce leaves

1 cup fresh or frozen kale leaves

1 cup fresh or frozen blueberries

¾ banana, peeled

Put all the ingredients in the blender in the order they are listed. Process on high speed until the mixture is smooth, adding water and/or ice as needed to achieve the desired consistency.

Protein: 26g • Calories: 337 • Dietary Fiber: 14g

Greens, Grapes, and Berries Smoothie

½ cup water

1 serving smoothie mix (pages 139–40) or 1 serving other protein
  powder

2 cups Swiss chard

2 cups fresh or frozen raspberries

1 cup seedless grapes

Put all the ingredients in the blender in the order they are listed. Process on high speed until the mixture is smooth, adding water and/or ice as needed to achieve the desired consistency.

Protein: 25g • Calories: 356 • Dietary Fiber: 23g

Green Tea–Berry Blend Smoothie

1 cup brewed and cooled unsweetened green tea

1 serving smoothie mix (pages 139–40) or 1 serving other protein powder

1 cup fresh or frozen spinach

1½ cups fresh or frozen blueberries

1¼ cups fresh or frozen raspberries

Put all the ingredients in the blender in the order they are listed. Process on high speed until the mixture is smooth, adding water and/or ice as needed to achieve the desired consistency.

Protein: 24g • Calories: 326 • Dietary Fiber: 21g

Living Green Smoothie

½ cup unsweetened coconut water

1 serving smoothie mix (pages 139–40) or 1 serving other protein powder

1 teaspoon fresh lemon juice

1 teaspoon grated ginger

1 cup fresh or frozen kale leaves

1 cup cucumber chunks

1½ pears, halved and cored

Put all the ingredients in the blender in the order they are listed. Process on high speed until the mixture is smooth, adding water and/or ice as needed to achieve the desired consistency.

Protein: 25g • Calories: 340 • Dietary Fiber: 17g

Orange-Cranberry-Cucumber Smoothie

½ cup water

½ cup fresh orange juice

1 serving smoothie mix (pages 139–40) or 1 serving other protein
  powder

1 cup fresh orange segments

1 cup fresh or frozen cranberries

1 cup cucumber chunks

2 packed cups mesclun salad mix

½ teaspoon finely grated orange zest (optional)

Put all the ingredients in the blender in the order they are listed. Process on high speed until the mixture is smooth, adding water and/or ice as needed to achieve the desired consistency.

Protein: 24g • Calories: 329 • Dietary Fiber: 17g

Orange Juiced-Up Smoothie

½ cup water

1 serving smoothie mix (pages 139–40) or 1 serving other protein powder

1 teaspoon fresh lemon juice

¼ cup fresh orange juice

2 cups fresh or frozen spinach

1 cup fresh orange segments

1 banana, peeled

Put all the ingredients in the blender in the order they are listed. Process on high speed until the mixture is smooth, adding water and/or ice as needed to achieve the desired consistency.

Protein: 25g • Calories: 343 • Dietary Fiber: 14g

Peachy Keen Smoothie

1 cup unsweetened almond milk

1 serving smoothie mix (pages 139–40) or 1 serving other protein powder

1 cup fresh or frozen kale leaves

1 cup sliced apricots

1 cup sliced peaches

1 teaspoon fresh ginger (optional)

1 teaspoon almond extract (optional)

Put all the ingredients in the blender in the order they are listed. Process on high speed until the mixture is smooth, adding water and/or ice as needed to achieve the desired consistency.

Protein: 27g • Calories: 324 • Dietary Fiber: 13g

Pineapple Dream Smoothie

½ cup water

1 serving smoothie mix (pages 139–40) or 1 serving other protein
    powder

2 cups fresh or frozen kale leaves

2 cups pineapple chunks

Put all the ingredients in the blender in the order they are listed. Process on high speed until the mixture is smooth, adding water and/or ice as needed to achieve the desired consistency.

Protein: 26g • Calories: 342 • Dietary Fiber: 12g

Raspberry-Orange Refresher

½ cup water

1 serving smoothie mix (pages 139–40) or 1 serving other protein
  powder

2 cups fresh or frozen spinach

1½ cups fresh or frozen raspberries

1 small orange, peeled and segmented

½ cup fresh orange juice

Put all the ingredients in the blender in the order they are listed. Process on high speed until the mixture is smooth, adding water and/or ice as needed to achieve the desired consistency.

Protein: 26g • Calories: 340 • Dietary Fiber: 22g

Spa Sipper Smoothie

- 1 cup unsweetened almond milk
- 1 serving smoothie mix (pages 139–40) or 1 serving other protein powder
- 1 cup cucumber chunks
- 2 cups fresh or frozen spinach
- ½ cup fresh or frozen mango cubes
- 1 banana, peeled

Put all the ingredients in the blender in the order they are listed. Process on high speed until the mixture is smooth, adding water and/or ice as needed to achieve the desired consistency.

Protein: 25g • Calories: 338 • Dietary Fiber: 13g

Spinach-Orange-Coriander Cooler

½ cup water

1 serving smoothie mix (pages 139–40) or 1 serving other protein powder

Juice of 1 lime

¼ cup coriander

2½ cups fresh or frozen spinach

1 cup fresh orange segments

1 cup fresh orange juice

Put all the ingredients in the blender in the order they are listed. Process on high speed until the mixture is smooth, adding water and/or ice as needed to achieve the desired consistency.

Protein: 25g • Calories: 336 • Dietary Fiber: 12g

Strawberry-Melon Magic Smoothie

½ cup nonfat milk

1 serving smoothie mix (pages 139–40) or 1 serving other protein powder

1 cup fresh or frozen spinach leaves

1¼ cups seedless watermelon cubes

2 cups fresh or frozen strawberries

Put all the ingredients in the blender in the order they are listed. Process on high speed until the mixture is smooth, adding water and/or ice as needed to achieve the desired consistency.

Protein: 28g • Calories: 315 • Dietary Fiber: 13g

Strawberry-Peach-Cucumber Cooler

½ cup water

1 serving smoothie mix (pages 139–40) or 1 serving other protein powder

1 teaspoon pure vanilla extract

1½ cups fresh or frozen strawberries

1½ cups fresh or frozen sliced peaches

1 cup cucumber chunks

2 tablespoons chopped fresh mint

1 cup packed mixed baby lettuce

Put all the ingredients in the blender in the order they are listed. Process on high speed until the mixture is smooth, adding water and/or ice as needed to achieve the desired consistency.

Protein: 25g • Calories: 311 • Dietary Fiber: 15g

Strawberry Sipper

½ cup water

1 serving smoothie mix (pages 139–40) or 1 serving other protein powder

2 teaspoons fresh lemon juice or orange juice

2½ cups fresh or frozen strawberries

½ cup fresh or frozen raspberries

1 kiwi fruit, sliced

1½ cups baby salad greens

Put all the ingredients in the blender in the order they are listed. Process on high speed until the mixture is smooth, adding water and/or ice as needed to achieve the desired consistency.

Protein: 25g • Calories: 324 • Dietary Fiber: 20g

Tropical Burst Smoothie

1 cup unsweetened coconut water

1 serving smoothie mix (pages 139–40) or 1 serving other protein powder

1 cup fresh or frozen spinach

1 cup fresh or frozen pineapple cubes

¾ cup fresh or frozen mango cubes

Put all the ingredients in the blender in the order they are listed. Process on high speed until the mixture is smooth, adding water and/or ice as needed to achieve the desired consistency.

Protein: 24g • Calories: 325 • Dietary Fiber: 13g

Walking on Sunshine Smoothie

½ cup water

1 serving smoothie mix (pages 139–40) or 1 serving other protein powder

1 cup unsweetened coconut water

1 cup fresh or frozen pineapple pieces, or well drained, if canned

½ cup fresh or frozen mango cubes

½ cup fresh or frozen raspberries

1 cup frozen chopped spinach

Put all the ingredients in the blender in the order they are listed. Process on high speed until the mixture is smooth, adding water and/or ice as needed to achieve the desired consistency.

Protein: 25g • Calories: 331 • Dietary Fiber: 16g

Winter Fresh Smoothie

½ cup water

1 serving smoothie mix (pages 139–40) or 1 serving other protein powder

1 tablespoon chopped fresh mint

¾ teaspoon finely grated orange zest

1 cup peeled orange segments

½ cup fresh or frozen cranberries

½ cup seedless red grapes

1 small apple, halved and cored

1½ cups packed baby spinach or frozen chopped spinach

Put all the ingredients in the blender in the order they are listed. Process on high speed until the mixture is smooth, adding water and/or ice as needed to achieve the desired consistency.

Protein: 24g • Calories: 334 • Dietary Fiber: 15g

HOT SUPERCHARGED SMOOTHIES

On crisp autumn and cool spring mornings as well as frigid winter days, a hot smoothie is much more appealing and comforting. Here are some hot SuperCharged Smoothies that will warm you up.

Caramel Apple Cider Smoothie

½ cup warm water

1 serving smoothie mix (pages 139–40) or 1 serving other protein powder

2½ small apples, cored and chopped

1 cup chopped cos lettuce leaves

2 teaspoons caramel extract

2 teaspoons vanilla extract

2 teaspoons ground cinnamon

Water, as needed

Put all the ingredients in a blender in the order listed. Process on high speed until the mixture is smooth, then pour into a saucepan and heat. Do not boil.

Protein: 22g • Calories: 336 • Dietary Fiber: 13g

Cocoa Warm-Up Smoothie

1 cup unsweetened almond milk, heated

1 serving smoothie mix (pages 139–40) or 1 serving other protein powder

¼ cup unsweetened cocoa powder

1 banana, peeled

2 teaspoons vanilla extract (optional)

Water, as needed

Put all the ingredients in a blender in the order listed. Process on high speed until the mixture is smooth, then pour into a saucepan and heat. Do not boil.

Protein: 26g • Calories: 326 • Dietary Fiber: 16g

Chamomile Chameleon Smoothie

1 cup brewed chamomile tea

1 serving smoothie mix (pages 139–40) or 1 serving other protein
  powder

1 cup sliced cucumber

2½ cups fresh or frozen raspberries

2 teaspoons agave nectar (optional)

Water, as needed

Put all the ingredients in a blender in the order listed. Process on high
speed until the mixture is smooth, then pour into a saucepan and
heat. Do not boil.

Protein: 24g • Calories: 318 • Dietary Fiber: 26g

Creamy Chai Smoothie

1 cup brewed unsweetened chai tea

½ cup nonfat milk

1 serving smoothie mix (pages 139–40) or 1 serving other protein
  powder

1 teaspoon ground cinnamon

1 teaspoon ground cloves

1 teaspoon ground nutmeg

1 cup chopped cos lettuce leaves

1½ bananas, peeled

Water, as needed

Put all the ingredients in a blender in the order listed. Process on high speed until the mixture is smooth, then pour into a saucepan and heat. Do not boil.

Protein: 27g • Calories: 344 • Dietary Fiber: 13g

Coffee-Cherry Warm-Up Smoothie

1 cup brewed coffee

½ cup nonfat milk

1 serving smoothie mix (pages 139–40) or 1 serving other protein powder

1 cup fresh or frozen spinach leaves

1 small carrot, peeled and chopped

1¼ cups pitted cherries

2 teaspoons agave nectar (optional)

Water, as needed

Put all the ingredients in a blender in the order listed. Process on high speed until the mixture is smooth, then pour into a saucepan and heat. Do not boil.

Protein: 28g • Calories: 334 • Dietary Fiber: 11g

Hot Cocoa Nut Smoothie

1 cup nonfat milk, warmed

1 serving smoothie mix (pages 139–40) or 1 serving other protein powder

1 tablespoon unsweetened cocoa powder

1 teaspoon coconut oil

1 cup sliced cucumber

½ carrot, peeled and sliced

1 orange, peeled and segmented

1 teaspoon vanilla extract (optional)

Water, as needed

Put all the ingredients in a blender in the order listed. Process on high speed until the mixture is smooth, then pour into a saucepan and heat. Do not boil.

Protein: 31g • Calories: 352 • Dietary Fiber: 12g

Meet Your Matcha Smoothie

1 cup heated nonfat milk

1 serving smoothie mix (pages 139–40) or 1 serving other protein powder

1 teaspoon matcha green tea powder

2 cups chopped cos lettuce leaves

1 banana, peeled

Water, as needed

Put all the ingredients in a blender in the order listed. Process on high speed until the mixture is smooth, then pour into a saucepan and heat. Do not boil.

Protein: 33g • Calories: 331 • Dietary Fiber: 10g

Raspberry Hot Chocolate Smoothie

1 cup nonfat milk, warmed

1 serving smoothie mix (pages 139–40) or 1 serving other protein powder

1 tablespoon unsweetened cocoa powder

1 cup chopped cos lettuce leaves

1½ cups fresh or frozen raspberries

1 teaspoon vanilla extract (optional)

Water, as needed

Put all the ingredients in a blender in the order listed. Process on high speed until the mixture is smooth, then pour into a saucepan and heat. Do not boil.

Protein: 32g • Calories: 324 • Dietary Fiber: 20g

SLEEPYTIME SUPERCHARGED SMOOTHIES

If falling and staying asleep are challenges for you, then try drinking one of these smoothies for dinner on all-smoothie days.

A Peachy Night's Sleep Smoothie

½ cup water

2 tablespoons tart cherry juice concentrate

1 serving smoothie mix (pages 139–40) or 1 serving other protein powder

1½ cups chopped spinach leaves

1 cup pitted cherries

1½ cup sliced peaches

Put all the ingredients in the blender in the order they are listed. Process on high speed until the mixture is smooth, adding water and/or ice as needed to achieve the desired consistency.

Protein: 25g • Calories: 324 • Dietary Fiber: 13g

Cherry-Almond Sleep Treat Smoothie

1½ cups unsweetened almond milk

2 tablespoons tart cherry juice concentrate

1 serving smoothie mix (pages 139–40) or 1 serving other protein powder

1 cup fresh or frozen kale leaves

1 banana, peeled

Put all the ingredients in the blender in the order they are listed. Process on high speed until the mixture is smooth, adding water and/or ice as needed to achieve the desired consistency.

Protein: 25g • Calories: 325 • Dietary Fiber: 11g

Cherry-Berry Dreamland Smoothie

½ cup water

2 tablespoons tart cherry juice concentrate

1 serving smoothie mix (pages 139–40) or 1 serving other protein
  powder

2 cups chopped spinach leaves

1 cup fresh or frozen strawberries

1½ cups pitted cherries

Put all the ingredients in the blender in the order they are listed. Process on high speed until the mixture is smooth, adding water and/or ice as needed to achieve the desired consistency.

Protein: 26g • Calories: 335 • Dietary Fiber: 15g

Citrus Sleeper Smoothie

½ cup water

2 tablespoons tart cherry juice concentrate

1 serving smoothie mix (pages 139–40) or 1 serving other protein powder

1 cup cucumber chunks

1 cup pitted cherries

1 cup fresh orange segments

Put all the ingredients in the blender in the order they are listed. Process on high speed until the mixture is smooth, adding water and/or ice as needed to achieve the desired consistency.

Protein: 24g • Calories: 325 • Dietary Fiber: 14g

CHAPTER 9

SuperCharged Soups

While SuperCharged Smoothies are delicious year-round, as the winter months approach sometimes you just need a filling and hearty soup! The Age-Defying Diet eliminates the guesswork and experimentation by providing you with simple SuperCharged Soup recipes that contain just as much nutritional protein and flavor as Super-Charged Smoothies do. These comforting and filling SuperCharged Soups, made with fresh or frozen vegetables, protein powder, and seasonings, are just the ticket when you want something warm on a cold day. Enjoy these SuperCharged Soups in place of SuperCharged Smoothies at breakfast, lunch, or dinner.

You can use an unflavored, sugar-free protein powder (see page 139); just be certain that each serving contains at least 20 grams of protein. Be sure to taste-test the protein powder you are using; some protein powders do not mix well or taste good in hot soups.

And like my tasty SuperCharged Smoothies, these SuperCharged Soups are sure to be a hit at your next gathering. Whether it's a holiday, a relative's birthday, or a dinner party, break out one of these delicious SuperCharged Soups and your guests will start to wonder how you've been managing to look so trim while eating rich and tasty soup!

SUPERCHARGED SOUP RECIPES

Asparagus Soup

Makes 2 servings

4 teaspoons extra-virgin olive oil

½ cup chopped onions

1 teaspoon crushed garlic

½ teaspoon salt

¼ teaspoon ground black pepper

1½ pounds asparagus, tough ends trimmed, stalks and tips cut into 1-inch pieces

8 teaspoons dry white wine (optional)

3 cups low-sodium chicken stock

3 tablespoons fresh lemon juice, to taste

2 servings protein mix (pages 139–40) or 2 servings other protein powder

Heat the oil in a medium pot over medium-high heat. Add the onions and cook, stirring, until soft, 2 to 2½ minutes. Add the garlic, salt, and pepper and cook, stirring, until the garlic is fragrant, about 30 seconds. Add the asparagus and cook, stirring, for 1 minute. Add the white wine, if using, and cook until it is nearly evaporated, 45 seconds to 1 minute. Add the chicken stock, stir well, and bring to the boil. Reduce the heat and simmer uncovered, stirring occasionally, until the asparagus is very tender and the mixture is slightly reduced, 12 to 15 minutes. Add lemon juice to taste.

Remove the soup from the heat and puree with a handheld blender, or in two batches in a food processor or blender. To serve, add 1 serving of protein powder for each 2-cup serving of soup, blending or whisking well to combine. Serve hot.

Per serving: Protein: 33g • Calories: 314 • Dietary Fiber: 13g

Broccoli-Spinach Soup

Makes 2 servings

5 teaspoons extra-virgin olive oil

¾ cup chopped onions

2 teaspoons crushed garlic

½ teaspoon salt

¼ teaspoon ground black pepper

¼ teaspoon ground nutmeg

3 cups frozen broccoli florets, thawed, or chopped fresh broccoli

2 (10-ounce) packages frozen chopped spinach, thawed, or
   3 cups packed fresh spinach

10 teaspoons dry white wine (optional)

3 cups low-sodium chicken stock

2 tablespoons fresh lemon juice, to taste

2 servings protein mix (pages 139–40) or 2 servings other protein
   powder

Heat the oil in a medium pot over medium-high heat. Add the onions and cook, stirring, until soft, 2 to 2½ minutes. Add the garlic, salt, pepper, and nutmeg and cook, stirring, until the garlic is fragrant, about 30 seconds. Add the broccoli and spinach and cook, stirring, until the spinach is wilted, 1 to 2 minutes. Add the white wine, if using, and cook until it is nearly evaporated, 45 seconds to 1 minute. Add the chicken stock, stir well, and bring to the boil. Reduce the heat and simmer uncovered, stirring occasionally, until the mixture is slightly reduced, 12 to 15 minutes. Add lemon juice to taste.

Remove the soup from the heat and puree with a handheld blender, or in two batches in a food processor or blender. To serve, add 1 serving of protein powder for each 2-cup serving of soup, blending or whisking well to combine. Serve hot.

Per serving: Protein: 30g • Calories: 318 • Dietary Fiber: 7g

Carrot, Peach, and Ginger Soup

Makes 2 servings

2 teaspoons extra-virgin olive oil

½ cup chopped onions

1 pound frozen sliced carrots, thawed, or about 2 cups chopped fresh carrots

5 teaspoons peeled and chopped fresh ginger

½ teaspoon salt

¼ teaspoon ground black pepper

1 cup frozen sliced peaches, thawed, or 1 cup fresh peeled, pitted, and sliced peaches

2¾ cups low-sodium chicken stock

2 tablespoons fresh orange juice, or to taste

2 servings protein mix (pages 139–40) or 2 servings other protein powder

Heat the oil in a medium pot over medium-high heat. Add the onions and cook, stirring, until soft, 2 to 2½ minutes. Add the carrots, ginger, salt, and pepper and cook, stirring, for 2 minutes. Add the peaches and stir to incorporate. Add the chicken stock, stir well, and bring to the boil. Reduce the heat and simmer uncovered, stirring occasionally, until the mixture is slightly reduced, about 15 minutes. Add orange juice to taste.

Remove the soup from the heat and puree with a handheld blender, or in two batches in a food processor or blender. To serve, add 1 serving of protein powder for each 2-cup serving of soup, blending or whisking well to combine. Serve hot.

Per serving: Protein: 28g • Calories: 322 • Dietary Fiber: 13g

Carrot, Pumpkin, and Apple Soup

Makes 2 servings

4 teaspoons extra-virgin olive oil

1½ cups frozen sliced carrots, thawed, or fresh peeled and sliced
   carrots

¾ cup chopped onions

½ teaspoon crushed garlic

2 apples, peeled, cored, and diced

½ teaspoon salt

¼ teaspoon ground black pepper

¼ teaspoon ground cinnamon

Pinch of ground nutmeg

Pinch of dried thyme

10 teaspoons dry white wine (optional)

1 cup 100% pure pumpkin puree (not pumpkin pie filling)

2¾ cups low-sodium chicken stock or vegetable stock

2 servings protein mix (pages 139–40) or 2 servings other protein
   powder

Heat the oil in a medium pot over medium-high heat. Add the carrots
and onions and cook, stirring, until soft, 2 to 2½ minutes. Add the garlic and cook, stirring, until fragrant, 30 seconds. Add the apples, salt,
pepper, cinnamon, nutmeg, and thyme and cook, stirring, for 30 seconds. Add the white wine, if using, and cook until it is nearly evaporated,
45 seconds to 1 minute. Add the pumpkin puree and chicken stock, stir
well, and bring to the boil. Reduce the heat and simmer uncovered, stirring occasionally, until the mixture is slightly reduced, about 15 minutes.

Remove the soup from the heat and puree with a handheld blender,
or in two batches in a food processor or blender. To serve, add 1 serving of protein powder for each 2-cup serving of soup, blending or
whisking well to combine. Serve hot.

Per serving: Protein: 27g • Calories: 342 • Dietary Fiber: 10g

Cauliflower and Roasted Garlic Soup

Makes 2 servings

5 teaspoons extra-virgin olive oil

½ cup chopped onions

½ cup chopped celery

1½ cups frozen sliced carrots, thawed and chopped, or fresh peeled and chopped carrots

½ teaspoon dried thyme

½ teaspoon salt

¼ teaspoon ground white or black pepper

2 cups frozen cauliflower florets, thawed, or 2 cups chopped fresh cauliflower florets

6 tablespoons Roasted Garlic (page 292) or 3 teaspoons crushed fresh garlic

3 cups low-sodium chicken stock

2 servings protein mix (pages 139–40) or 2 servings other protein powder

Heat the oil in a medium pot over medium-high heat. Add the onions, celery, carrots, thyme, salt, and pepper and cook, stirring, until the vegetables are soft, 3 minutes. (If you're using fresh garlic, add it now and sauté until fragrant, about 30 seconds.) Add the cauliflower and cook, stirring, until softened, 2 to 3 minutes. Add the roasted garlic and stir to incorporate. Add the chicken stock, stir well, and bring to the boil. Reduce the heat and simmer uncovered, stirring occasionally, until the mixture is slightly reduced, 12 to 15 minutes.

Remove the soup from the heat and puree with a handheld blender, or in two batches in a food processor or blender. To serve, add 1 serving of protein powder for each 2-cup serving of soup.

Per serving: Protein: 29g • Calories: 325 • Dietary Fiber: 11g

Creamy Broccoli Soup

Makes 2 servings

5 teaspoons extra-virgin olive oil

¾ cup chopped onions

1 teaspoon crushed garlic

½ teaspoon dried thyme

½ teaspoon salt

¼ teaspoon ground black pepper

1 (1-pound) bag frozen broccoli florets, thawed, or about
    2⅓ cups chopped fresh broccoli

10 teaspoons dry white wine (optional)

3 cups chicken stock

1½ tablespoons fresh lemon juice, to taste

2 servings protein mix (pages 139–40) or 2 servings other protein
    powder

Heat the oil in a medium pot over medium-high heat. Add the onions
and cook, stirring, until soft, 3 minutes. Add the garlic, thyme, salt,
and pepper and cook, stirring, until the garlic is fragrant, about
30 seconds. Add the broccoli and cook, stirring, until softened, 2 to
4 minutes. Add the white wine, if using, and cook until it is nearly
evaporated, 45 seconds to 1 minute. Add the chicken stock, stir well,
and bring to the boil. Reduce the heat and simmer uncovered, stirring occasionally, until the mixture is slightly reduced, about 15 minutes. Add lemon juice to taste.

Remove the soup from the heat and puree with a handheld blender,
or in two batches in a food processor or blender. To serve, add 1 serving of protein powder for each 2-cup serving of soup, blending or
whisking well to combine. Serve hot.

Per serving: Protein: 33g • Calories: 338 • Dietary Fiber: 6g

Creamy Mushroom Soup

Makes 2 servings

4 teaspoons extra-virgin olive oil

¾ cup chopped onions

½ cup chopped celery

½ teaspoon crushed garlic

½ teaspoon salt

¼ teaspoon ground black pepper

1½ teaspoons chopped fresh thyme or ½ teaspoon dried thyme

2 pounds button mushrooms, sliced

10 teaspoons dry white wine (optional)

4 cups low-sodium chicken stock or water

2 servings protein mix (pages 139–40) or 2 servings other protein powder

Heat the oil in a medium pot over medium-high heat. Add the onions and celery and cook, stirring, until soft, about 3 minutes. Add the garlic, salt, pepper, and thyme and cook, stirring, until the garlic is fragrant, about 30 seconds. Add the mushrooms and cook, stirring, until the mushrooms are wilted and give off their liquid, 6 to 7 minutes. Add the white wine, if using, and cook until it is nearly evaporated, 45 seconds to 1 minute. Add the chicken stock, stir well, and bring to the boil. Reduce the heat and simmer uncovered, stirring occasionally, until the mixture is slightly reduced, about 15 minutes.

Remove the soup from the heat and puree with a handheld blender, or in two batches in a food processor or blender. To serve, add 1 serving of protein powder for each serving of soup, blending or whisking well to combine. Serve hot.

Per serving: Protein: 34g • Calories: 313 • Dietary Fiber: 9g

Curried Courette-Cauliflower Soup

Makes 2 servings

5 teaspoons extra-virgin olive oil

½ cup chopped onions

½ teaspoon crushed garlic

1 teaspoon curry powder

½ teaspoon salt

Pinch of cayenne

12 ounces courgettes, trimmed and roughly chopped (about 1½ cups)

1½ cups frozen cauliflower florets, or 1½ cups trimmed fresh cauliflower florets

4 cups low-sodium chicken stock or vegetable stock

2 servings protein mix (pages 139–40) or 2 servings other protein powder

⅔ teaspoon sliced spring onions, for garnish

Heat the oil in a medium pot over medium-high heat. Add the onions and cook, stirring, until soft, 2 to 2½ minutes. Add the garlic, stir, and cook for 5 seconds. Add the curry powder, salt, and cayenne and cook, stirring, until the garlic and curry are fragrant, 20 seconds. Add the courgette and cauliflower and cook, stirring, until the vegetables are just soft and giving off their liquid, 2 to 3 minutes. Add the chicken stock, stir well, and bring to the boil. Reduce the heat and simmer uncovered, stirring occasionally, until the vegetables are very tender and the mixture is slightly reduced, about 15 minutes.

Remove the soup from the heat and puree with a handheld blender, or in two batches in a food processor or blender. To serve, add 1 serving of protein powder for each 2-cup serving of soup, blending or whisking well to combine. Serve hot, garnished with spring onions.

Per serving: Protein: 33g • Calories: 315 • Dietary Fiber: 10g

Kale, Spinach, and Tomato Soup

Makes 2 servings

5 teaspoons extra-virgin olive oil

½ cup chopped onions

¼ cup frozen sliced carrots, thawed, or fresh peeled and sliced carrots

½ teaspoon crushed garlic

½ teaspoon salt

¼ teaspoon crushed red pepper

1 (14½-ounce) can chopped tomatoes and their juice

1 cup frozen chopped kale or mustard greens, thawed, or 2 cups chopped fresh kale leaves

1 cup frozen chopped spinach, thawed

1 tablespoon chopped fresh basil or 1 teaspoon dried basil

1 teaspoon chopped fresh oregano or ¼ teaspoon dried oregano

4 cups low-sodium chicken stock or vegetable stock

2 servings protein mix (pages 139–40) or 2 servings other protein powder

Heat the oil in a medium pot over medium-high heat. Add the onions and carrots and cook, stirring, until soft, 2 to 2½ minutes. Add the garlic, salt, and red pepper, stir, and cook until the garlic is fragrant, 30 seconds. Add the tomatoes, kale, spinach, basil, and oregano and cook, stirring, until well combined and the vegetables start to give off their liquid, 1 to 2 minutes. Add the chicken stock, stir well, and bring to the boil. Reduce the heat and simmer uncovered, stirring occasionally, until the vegetables are very tender and the mixture is slightly reduced, about 5 minutes.

Remove the soup from the heat and puree with a handheld blender, or in two batches in a food processor or blender. To serve, add 1 serving of protein powder for each 2-cup serving of soup, blending or whisking well to combine.

Per serving: Protein: 31g • Calories: 323 • Dietary Fiber: 10g

Lentil, Tomato, and Spinach Soup

Makes 2 servings

1 teaspoon extra-virgin olive oil

½ cup chopped celery

¼ cup chopped onions

½ teaspoon crushed garlic

½ teaspoon salt

¼ teaspoon crushed red pepper

1 (12 ounce) can chopped tomatoes and their juice

1 cup frozen chopped spinach, thawed, or 1 cup frozen mustard greens, thawed

4 teaspoons chopped fresh basil or 1¼ teaspoons dried basil

1 teaspoon chopped fresh oregano or ¼ teaspoon dried oregano

½ cup green, brown, or red lentils

2 cups canned low-sodium chicken stock or vegetable stock

½–1½ cups water, as needed

2 servings protein mix (pages 139–40) or 2 servings other protein powder

Heat the oil in a medium pot over medium-high heat. Add the celery and onions and cook, stirring, until soft, 3 to 3½ minutes. Add the garlic, salt, and red pepper, stir, and cook until the garlic is fragrant, 30 seconds. Add the tomatoes, spinach or mustard greens, basil, and oregano and cook, stirring, until well combined and starting to give off their liquid, 1 to 2 minutes. Add the lentils and cook, stirring, for 20 seconds. Add the chicken stock, stir well, and bring to the boil. Reduce the heat and simmer uncovered, stirring occasionally, until the vegetables are very tender and the lentils are tender and the mixture is slightly reduced, 20 to 30 minutes, adding water as needed for a thinner consistency.

Remove the soup from the heat and puree with a handheld blender, or in two batches in a food processor or blender. To serve, add 1 serving of protein powder for each 2-cup serving of soup, blending or whisking well to combine.

Per serving: Protein: 38g • Calories: 367 • Dietary Fiber: 23g

Parsnip, Turnip, and Pear Soup

Makes 2 servings

2 teaspoons extra-virgin olive oil

½ cup chopped onions

1½ cups peeled and chopped parsnips

1 cup peeled and chopped turnips

½ teaspoon salt

¼ teaspoon freshly ground pepper

Pinch of cayenne

¼ teaspoon ground cinnamon

Pinch of ground allspice

1 cup peeled, cored, and chopped pears (about 2 large)

3¼ cups low-sodium chicken stock or vegetable stock

2 servings protein mix (pages 139–40) or 2 servings other protein
   powder

Heat the oil in a medium pot over medium-high heat. Add the onions and cook, stirring, until soft, 2 minutes. Add the parsnips, turnips, salt, pepper, cayenne, cinnamon, and allspice and cook, stirring, until the vegetables are starting to color and soften, about 5 minutes. Add the pears and stir to incorporate. Add the chicken stock, stir well, and bring to the boil. Reduce the heat and simmer uncovered, stirring occasionally, until the vegetables are tender and the mixture is slightly reduced, 20 to 30 minutes.

Remove the soup from the heat and puree with a handheld blender, or in two batches in a food processor or blender. To serve, add 1 serving of protein powder for each 2-cup serving of soup, blending or whisking well to combine. Serve hot.

Per serving: Protein: 28g • Calories: 327 • Dietary Fiber: 14g

Roasted Red and Yellow Pepper Soup

While a combination of red and yellow peppers makes a lovely soup, feel free to use peppers all of one color.

Makes 2 servings

4 teaspoons vegetable oil

½ cup chopped onions

½ teaspoon crushed garlic

½ teaspoon salt

¼ teaspoon freshly ground black pepper

2 Roasted Red Peppers (page 254)

2 Roasted Yellow Peppers (page 254)

2 tablespoons dry white wine (optional)

½ cup peeled and roughly chopped fresh orange segments

½ cup canned chopped tomatoes and their juice

¼ cup fresh orange juice

1½ teaspoons finely grated orange zest

1 tablespoon chopped fresh basil leaves or 1 teaspoon
    dried basil

4 cups low-sodium chicken stock or vegetable stock

2 servings protein mix (pages 139–40) or 2 servings other protein
    powder

Heat the oil in a large pot over medium-high heat. Add the onions and cook, stirring, until soft, 2 to 2½ minutes. Add the garlic, salt, and pepper and cook, stirring, until the garlic is fragrant, about 30 seconds. Add the peppers and their juice and cook, stirring, for 1 minute. Add the white wine, if using, and cook until it is nearly evaporated, 45 seconds to 1 minute. Add the oranges, tomatoes and their juice, orange juice, orange zest, and basil and cook, stirring, until the mixture starts to thicken, 2 to 3 minutes. Add the chicken stock, stir well, and bring to the boil. Reduce the heat and simmer uncovered, stirring occasionally, until the mixture is slightly reduced, 12 to 15 minutes.

Remove the soup from the heat and puree with a handheld blender, or in two batches in a food processor. To serve, add 1 serving of protein powder for each serving of soup, blending or whisking well to combine. Serve hot.

Per serving: Protein: 24g • Calories: 329 • Dietary Fiber: 11g

Southwestern Soup

Makes 2 servings

4 teaspoons extra-virgin olive oil

½ cup chopped onions

2 poblano peppers, roasted, peeled, seeded, and chopped according to the instructions for Roasted Peppers (page 254)

½ cup chopped Roasted Red and Yellow Peppers (page 257), or ½ cup chopped fresh red or yellow peppers

1 tablespoon Roasted Garlic (page 292) or ½ teaspoon crushed fresh garlic

1 teaspoon seeded and minced jalapeño

½ teaspoon salt

½ teaspoon ground cumin

⅛ teaspoon ground coriander

1 (14½-ounce) can chopped tomatoes and their juice

1 cup frozen chopped spinach, thawed

2 tablespoons chopped fresh coriander, plus additional for garnish if desired

1¼ cups low-sodium chicken stock or vegetable stock

1–2 tablespoons fresh lime juice, to taste

2 servings protein mix (pages 139–40) or 2 servings other protein powder

Heat the oil in a medium pot over medium-high heat. Add the onions and cook, stirring, until soft, 2 to 2½ minutes. (If you are adding fresh peppers instead of roasted, cook them with the onions.) Add the roasted poblanos, peppers, garlic, jalapeño, salt, cumin, and ground coriander, stir, and cook for 45 seconds. Add the tomatoes, spinach, and the 2 tablespoons of fresh coriander and cook, stirring, until well combined and starting to give off their liquid, 1 to 2 minutes. Add the chicken stock, stir well, and bring to the boil. Reduce the heat and simmer uncovered, stirring occasionally, until the vegetables are tender and the mixture is slightly reduced, 10 to 15 minutes. Stir in lime juice to taste.

Remove the soup from the heat and puree with a handheld blender, or in two batches in a food processor or blender. To serve, add 1 serving of protein powder for each 2-cup serving of soup, blending or whisking well to combine.

Per serving: Protein: 29g • Calories: 323 • Dietary Fiber: 16g

Tomato-Herb Soup

This soup brings the taste of summer into your kitchen, even on the coldest winter day!

Makes 2 servings

4 teaspoons vegetable oil

¾ cup chopped onions

½ cup chopped celery

¾ teaspoon crushed garlic

¼ teaspoon salt

¼ teaspoon freshly ground black pepper

Pinch of cayenne

1 (14½-ounce) can passata

1 (14½-ounce) can chopped tomatoes and their juice

1 tablespoon chopped fresh basil leaves or 1 teaspoon dried basil

2 teaspoons chopped fresh oregano leaves or ¾ teaspoon dried oregano

3 cups low-sodium chicken stock or water

2 servings protein mix (pages 139–40) or 2 servings other protein powder

Heat the oil in a large pot over medium-high heat. Add the onions and celery and cook, stirring, until soft, about 3 minutes. Add the garlic, salt, pepper, and cayenne and cook, stirring, until the garlic is fragrant, about 30 seconds. Add the passata, basil, and oregano and stir to combine. Add the chicken stock, stir well, and bring to the boil. Reduce the heat and simmer uncovered, stirring occasionally, until the mixture is slightly reduced, 12 to 15 minutes.

Remove the soup from the heat and puree with a handheld blender, or in two batches in a food processor. To serve, add 1 serving of protein powder for each serving of soup, blending or whisking well to combine. Serve hot.

Per serving: Protein: 29g • Calories: 317 • Dietary Fiber: 11g

Courgette-Spinach Soup

Makes 2 servings

5 teaspoons extra-virgin olive oil

½ cup chopped onions

1 teaspoon crushed garlic

½ teaspoon salt

¼ teaspoon ground black pepper

1 pound courgettes, trimmed and roughly chopped (about 2½ cups)

4 cups low-sodium chicken stock or vegetable stock

1½ cups packed frozen spinach

1 tablespoon chopped parsley leaves

2 teaspoons finely grated lemon zest

2 servings protein mix (pages 139–40) or 2 servings other protein powder

Heat the oil in a medium pot over medium-high heat. Add the onions and cook, stirring, until soft, 2 to 2½ minutes. Add the garlic, salt, and pepper and cook, stirring, until the garlic is fragrant, about 30 seconds. Add the courgettes and cook, stirring, until they give off their liquid and are soft but still bright green and not completely dry, 4 to 5 minutes. Add the chicken stock, stir well, and bring to the boil. Reduce the heat and simmer uncovered, stirring occasionally, for 8 minutes. Add the spinach, parsley, and lemon zest, stir, and cook until the mixture is slightly reduced, about 5 minutes.

Remove the soup from the heat and puree with a handheld blender, or in two batches in a food processor or blender. To serve, add 1 serving of protein powder for each 2-cup serving of soup, blending or whisking well to combine. Serve hot.

Per serving: Protein: 34g • Calories: 314 • Dietary Fiber: 9g

CHAPTER 10

Whole-Food Meal Recipes

While drinking satisfying, delicious protein SuperCharged Smoothies is essential when it comes to boosting your metabolism and knocking off those pounds, eating healthy whole meals is just as important. Here are quick-and-easy recipes for those all-important protein main courses—chicken breasts, steak, pork tenderloin, shrimp, and more. Each recipe makes four servings, so you can serve them to your family, refrigerate for leftovers, or freeze extra portions for future meals.

When it comes to vegetables, I offer a number of different techniques for cooking them. There's a section for whole grains and recipes for sauces and condiments. These can be used with the main course, vegetable, and whole-grain recipes and snacks. Drizzle a tablespoon or two of Orange-Mint Yogurt Sauce over some steamed asparagus. Top Turkey Meat Loaf with Tomato Sauce. Stir some Pesto into cooked Quinoa. By mixing and matching these recipes, you'll never be bored. You can always add fresh herbs and spices to satisfy those taste buds of yours, whether you've got a zest for heavy spice or you just need a little dash of something to make your meal right.

Finally, there are some dessert recipes included to finish your meal, but know that you can always enjoy some fresh fruit, and you can find ready-made desserts on my website DrApovian.com.

What If There's No Time to Make a Whole-Food Meal?

Many times when my patients have come to me, one of their biggest issues is trying to figure out what to eat and how to make it. While I take the riddles and guesswork out for you with these delicious whole-food meal recipes that contain all the right ingredients to give you that slim figure you've been wanting, sometimes you're too busy or can't bother to cook that night. And on those nights, there are some frozen foods that will make eating easy, enjoyable, and healthy.

Most supermarkets now offer a variety of healthy ready-made meal options. For frozen whole-food meals, use these guidelines: Your frozen dinners should have 150 to 350 calories, 15 grams protein, 3 grams fiber, and no more than 600 milligrams sodium. (I recommend few frozen dinners, because most of them contain too much sodium.) If you do choose one of these, accompany it with a SuperCharged Smoothie to make certain you're consuming enough protein and calories.

BEEF

Sirloin Steaks with Mushroom Sauce

Nothing beats a steak with a rich mushroom sauce for a meal. Use the leanest meat you can find and trim off all the fat before cooking.

Makes 4 servings

4 sirloin steaks, 6 ounces each, at room temperature and patted dry

½ teaspoon salt

1¼ teaspoons ground black pepper, divided

1¼ teaspoons extra-virgin olive oil, divided

¼ cup chopped shallots or onions

¼ teaspoon chopped fresh thyme, or pinch of dried thyme

1 cup dry red wine

½ cup low-sodium beef or chicken stock

8 ounces button mushrooms, wiped clean, stems trimmed, and sliced ¼ inch thick

¾ teaspoon fresh tarragon or ¼ teaspoon dried tarragon

Preheat the oven to 350°F.

Season both sides of the steaks with salt and 1 teaspoon of the pepper.

Heat 1 teaspoon of the oil in a large, ovenproof, nonstick skillet over medium-high heat. Add the steaks to the pan and sear, 1½ to 2 minutes. Turn and cook for 1 minute on the second side. Remove the pan from the heat. Transfer the steaks to an oven rack set over a pan or a large baking dish and roast until the meat is cooked to your desired temperature, 5 to 10 minutes, depending upon the size and thickness.

As you prepare the sauce, check the meat periodically and remove it from the oven when done. Let it rest on a clean plate, tenting it to keep it warm as you finish the sauce. To make the sauce, return the cooking skillet to medium-high heat. To the fat in the pan, add the remaining ¼ teaspoon oil, the shallots, thyme, and ¼ teaspoon pepper and cook until the shallots are fragrant and soft, about 1½ to 2 minutes. Add the wine, bring to a simmer, and cook, stirring to remove any browned bits remaining on the bottom of the pan, until the liquid is reduced by half. Add the stock, bring to the boil, and cook until reduced by half, 1½ to 2 minutes. Add the mushrooms, lower the heat, and simmer until the mushrooms are tender, about 2 minutes. Remove the pan from the heat. Stir in the tarragon and adjust the seasoning to taste. Place one steak on each of four large plates; spoon the sauce over the steaks. Serve immediately.

Per serving: Protein: 37g • Calories: 342 • Dietary Fiber: 1g

Serve with unlimited salad, fruit, and nonstarchy vegetables and ½ cup grains.

Beef and Vegetable Kebabs

For successful kebabs, cook the meat and the vegetable kebabs separately, since the vegetables often cook faster than the meat. If you're using wooden skewers, soak them in water for 20 to 30 minutes so they don't burn. Kebabs can also be made in a grill pan.

Makes 4 servings

1½ pounds beef sirloin tips, cut into 2-inch cubes, divided into 6-ounce servings

1 cup fresh orange juice

1 tablespoon red wine vinegar

1 tablespoon dry red wine

1 tablespoon Worcestershire sauce

2 teaspoons soy sauce

2 cloves garlic, peeled and crushed

1 teaspoon ground black pepper

8 ounces button mushrooms, wiped clean and halved

1 large red pepper, seeded and cored, cut into 2-inch wedges

1 large red onion, cut into 2-inch wedges

1 medium courgette, cut into ¾-inch slices

Olive oil cooking spray

Place the meat in a large, resealable plastic bag.

To make the marinade, whisk together the orange juice, vinegar, wine, Worcestershire sauce, soy sauce, garlic, and black pepper in a small bowl. Pour the mixture into the bag with the meat and tightly seal. Turn the bag to coat the meat evenly and place inside a baking dish in the refrigerator for at least 3 and up to 6 hours, turning occasionally.

Preheat a grill to medium-high. If you're using bamboo skewers, place them in a large baking dish, cover with water and soak for 30 minutes.

Transfer the beef cubes from the marinade to a baking dish and pat dry. Thread the meat onto the skewers. Then thread vegetables onto separate skewers. Spray the skewers and the grill lightly with the cooking spray. Place the kebabs on the grill and cook, turning occasionally, until the meat reaches your desired temperature and the vegetables are charred and cooked through, 8 to 10 minutes. Remove the kebabs from the grill and serve hot.

Per serving: Protein: 38g • Calories: 356 • Dietary Fiber: 3g

Serve with unlimited salad, fruit, and nonstarchy vegetables and ½ cup grains.

CHICKEN

Chicken Breasts Baked in Foil Packets

When you need cooked chicken for a salad or dinner, this quick and simple method of oven poaching in foil packets is the one to use. You can enjoy these breasts as soon as they're cooked, or chop or shred the meat to use in other recipes. Vary the vegetables and flavors by substituting green beans or sliced courgette, or lemon slices and two bay leaves.

Makes 4 servings

- 1 cup chopped carrots
- 1 cup chopped celery
- 2 tablespoons chopped parsley, divided
- 4 boneless, skinless chicken breasts (6 ounces each)
- 1 teaspoon salt
- ½ teaspoon ground black pepper
- 1 cup low-sodium chicken stock or water

Preheat the oven to 350°F. Cut 4 sheets of aluminum foil, approximately 18 x 12 inches. Divide the vegetables and 1 tablespoon parsley among the 4 pieces of foil. Lay 1 chicken breast on top of the vegetables and season lightly with salt and pepper. Divide and spoon the chicken stock or water around each chicken breast. Close each package by drawing the sides of the foil packet together to seal well. Place the packets on a baking sheet and bake for 30 to 36 minutes, depending upon the size of the breasts. Remove the pan from the oven and carefully unwrap the foil packet. Let the chicken rest until it is cool enough to chop or shred, or serve immediately.

Per serving: Protein: 40g • Calories: 206 • Dietary Fiber: 1g

Pan-Cooked Chicken Breasts

This simple method of starting your chicken in a pan and then finishing it in the oven can also be used to cook other meats, including lean pork chops and steaks. Larger and thicker cuts of meat will take longer to cook; adjust your cooking times accordingly.

Serve your chicken hot, topped with Lemon-Artichoke Sauce (page 283) or homemade Tomato Sauce (page 287). Or take leftovers to work and serve chilled on top of a big green salad with Pico de Gallo (page 290) or Mango Salsa (page 289).

Makes 4 servings

4 boneless, skinless chicken breasts (6 ounces each)

½ teaspoon salt

1 teaspoon ground black pepper

1 teaspoon extra-virgin olive oil

Preheat the oven to 350°F.

Season both sides of the chicken with salt and pepper.

Heat the oil in a large nonstick skillet over medium-high heat. Add the chicken to the pan and sear for 2 minutes. Turn and cook for 1 minute on the second side. Remove the pan from the heat. Transfer the chicken to a baking dish and roast until the chicken is cooked through, 10 to 15 minutes.

Per serving: Protein: 39g • Calories: 195 • Dietary Fiber: 0g

Serve with unlimited salad, fruit, and nonstarchy vegetables and ½ cup grains.

Chicken Breasts Stuffed with Ricotta Creamed Spinach

Skinless, boneless chicken breasts are filled with spinach and ricotta cheese, and then baked. To make this a complete Italian meal, serve with ½ cup of Whole Wheat Pasta (page 263), a few tablespoons of Tomato Sauce (page 287), and some steamed broccoli.

Makes 4 servings

4 boneless, skinless chicken breasts (6 ounces each)

3–4 tablespoons Ricotta Creamed Spinach (page 251)

¾ teaspoon salt

¼ teaspoon ground black pepper

1 teaspoon vegetable oil

1⅓ cups Tomato Sauce (page 287) (optional)

4 teaspoons freshly grated Parmigiano-Reggiano cheese (optional)

Preheat the oven to 350°F. Insert a small sharp knife into the thick side of each chicken breast and make a pocket about 3 inches long and 1½ to 2 inches deep. Stuff each breast with 2½ teaspoons to 1 tablespoon of the spinach mixture and close the pocket with a toothpick. Season both sides of the chicken with the salt and pepper.

Heat the oil in a large nonstick, ovenproof skillet over medium-high heat. Add the chicken to the pan and sear for 2 minutes. Turn, transfer the skillet to the oven, and roast until the chicken is cooked through, 10 to 15 minutes. Meanwhile, heat the sauce in a small saucepan over medium heat, stirring occasionally. Place one chicken breast on each of four large plates. Remove the toothpicks. If desired, spoon ⅓ cup of the sauce over each serving, and sprinkle with cheese. Serve immediately.

Per serving: Protein: 42g • Calories: 239 • Dietary Fiber: 0g

Serve with unlimited salad, fruit, and nonstarchy vegetables and ½ cup grains or pasta.

Chicken with Red Grapes

The longer you cook this sauce, the more it will reduce, and also the more intense a flavor the grapes will develop.

Makes 4 servings

4 boneless, skinless chicken breasts (6 ounces each)

1¼ teaspoons ground black pepper, divided

⅝ teaspoon salt, divided

1 teaspoon extra-virgin olive oil

2 tablespoons chopped shallots or onions

2 tablespoons dry white wine

1 teaspoon fresh lemon juice

¾ cup low-sodium chicken stock

¼ teaspoon chopped fresh thyme or pinch of dried thyme

1½ cups halved seedless red grapes

1 teaspoon chopped fresh parsley

Preheat the oven to 350°F. Season both sides of the chicken with 1 teaspoon of the pepper and ½ teaspoon of the salt.

Heat the oil in a large nonstick skillet over medium-high heat. Add the chicken to the pan and sear for 2 minutes. Turn and cook for 1 minute on the second side. Remove the pan from the heat. Transfer the chicken to a baking dish and roast until the chicken is cooked through, 10 to 15 minutes. Return the pan to medium heat. Add the shallots or onions and remaining ¼ teaspoon pepper and ⅛ teaspoon salt to the browned bits remaining in the pan. Cook, stirring, with a wooden spoon, until the onions are soft, 1 to 1½ minutes. Add the wine and lemon juice and cook until nearly evaporated, about 30 seconds. Add the stock and thyme and stir to incorporate. Increase the heat, bring to a simmer, and cook until the liquid begins to reduce, 1 to 2 minutes. Add the grapes and cook until they are softened and the sauce is reduced by half, 1½ to 2½ minutes. Remove from the heat and stir in the parsley. Place one chicken breast on each of four large plates. Spoon the sauce and grapes over each chicken breast and serve immediately.

Per serving: Protein: 40g • Calories: 244 • Dietary Fiber: 1g

Serve with unlimited salad, fruit, and nonstarchy vegetables and ½ cup grains.

Garlic-Lemon Chicken

Make this dish with chicken thighs; chicken breasts will dry out. Cooking the garlic with the thighs and other ingredients mellows its flavor and softens its texture. Round out your meal by serving the extra sauce on top of Brown Rice (page 258) or Whole Wheat Pasta (page 263), or plain Courgette Noodles (page 255).

Makes 4 servings

1 (1½-pound) package boneless, skinless chicken thighs

¾ teaspoon salt

1 teaspoon ground black pepper

2 teaspoons extra-virgin olive oil

1½ teaspoons chopped garlic

2 tablespoons white wine

6 large whole cloves garlic, peeled, and halved if very large (about 2 tablespoons)

2 tablespoons fresh lemon juice

1 teaspoon fresh lemon zest

2 teaspoons chopped fresh oregano or ¾ teaspoon dried oregano

2 teaspoons chopped fresh parsley, plus 1 tablespoon for garnish

⅔ cup low-sodium chicken stock

Preheat the oven to 350°F. Season the chicken on both sides with the salt and pepper.

Heat a large, heavy, nonstick, ovenproof skillet over medium heat. Add the oil and swirl to evenly coat the bottom of the pan. When the oil is hot, add the chicken—be careful not to overcrowd or the meat will steam—and sear on the first side, 2 minutes. Turn the thighs and sear on the second side for 2 minutes. Remove thighs to a plate and tent with foil while you prepare the sauce. Add the chopped garlic to the pan and cook, stirring, for 30 seconds. Add the white wine, stir, and cook for 20 to 30 seconds. Add the whole garlic cloves, lemon juice, and lemon zest and cook for 30 seconds. Add the herbs, stir, and add the chicken stock. Return thighs to the pan along with accumulated juices. Baste the thighs with the sauce. Bring the stock to the boil, cover, place the pan in the oven, and bake for 15 minutes. Remove the cover and bake for 5 minutes more.

Remove the pan from the oven and divide the chicken and sauce among four plates. Serve immediately, garnished with parsley. (If you'd like a thicker sauce, remove the thighs from the pan and cover to keep warm. Place the pan over medium-high heat and reduce the sauce to your desired thickness. Serve hot.)

Per serving: Protein: 34g • Calories: 235 • Dietary Fiber: 0g

Serve with unlimited salad, fruit, and nonstarchy vegetables and ½ cup grains.

TURKEY

Roasted Turkey Breast

Fresh herbs are essential in this recipe, as their natural oils provide the most flavor. Serve hot turkey slices plain or with some Brown Rice (page 258), and a pile of Roasted Vegetables (page 246). Any leftovers can be cubed and used in salads—or serve them cold in a salad topped with Mango Salsa (page 289).

Makes 4 servings

1 (24-ounce) boneless, skinless turkey breast half, tied with
  butcher's twine
1 tablespoon chopped fresh parsley
1 tablespoon chopped fresh rosemary
1 tablespoon chopped fresh sage
1 tablespoon extra-virgin olive oil
1 teaspoon grated lemon zest
½ teaspoon salt
½ teaspoon ground black pepper

Preheat the oven to 400°F. Place the meat in a large baking dish and let it come to room temperature, about 20 minutes.

Combine the remaining ingredients in a small bowl, mixing well with a fork, to make a paste. Rub the turkey with the herb mixture on both sides. Place in the oven and roast for 20 minutes. Reduce the temperature to 325°F and cook until the meat is cooked through, or until an instant-read thermometer inserted into the thickest part of the breast registers 165°F, about 1 hour. Transfer the turkey to a cutting board to rest for 20 to 30 minutes. Remove the twine and slice to serve. (The turkey will keep, refrigerated and tightly wrapped, for up to 5 days. Or you can freeze the sliced turkey in resealable freezer bags.)

Per serving: Protein: 37g • Calories: 295 • Dietary Fiber: 0g

Open-Faced Turkey-Portobello Burgers

Meaty, roasted portobello mushroom halves are used in place of buns to make open-faced burgers. As with the Turkey Meat Loaf (page 225), these burgers must be cooked "low and slow" until well done. Top them with Tomato Sauce (page 287), or Mayonnaise (page 282) and a slather of your favorite mustard.

Makes 4 burgers

- 4 portobello mushroom caps, stems removed, wiped clean with a damp towel
- 1 teaspoon plus 1½ teaspoons extra-virgin olive oil
- ¼ teaspoon plus ½ teaspoon salt
- ¼ teaspoon plus ¼ teaspoon ground black pepper
- 1 pound lean minced turkey
- 4 teaspoons sliced spring onions, green tops only
- 1 teaspoon chopped fresh oregano or ¼ teaspoon dried oregano
- ½ teaspoon crushed red pepper
- 2 teaspoons finely grated lemon zest
- 1 medium tomato, thinly sliced (optional)
- ¾ cup very thinly sliced sweet onions (optional)
- Condiments of choice, such as Tomato Sauce (page 287), Mayonnaise (page 282), or Dijon or yellow mustard

Preheat the oven to 400°F. Line a baking sheet with aluminum foil.

Gently scrape the gills from the inside of the mushrooms using a teaspoon. Lightly brush the top of each mushroom with ¼ teaspoon of the oil and season with a pinch of the salt and pepper. Place top-side down (gill-side up) on the baking sheet and roast until they give off their liquid and are tender, about 15 minutes. Turn the mushrooms and roast until they are dry, 3 to 5 minutes. Remove from the oven and let rest.

Combine the turkey, spring onions, oregano, red pepper, zest, and remaining ½ teaspoon salt and ¼ teaspoon black pepper in a large bowl. Mix with your fingers or a rubber spatula until well combined. Form into patties of the proper weight for your nutritional requirements.

Heat the remaining 1½ teaspoons oil in a large, heavy, nonstick skillet over medium-high heat. Add the patties and reduce the heat to medium. Cook uncovered for 5 minutes. Turn the patties and cook until the meat is completely cooked through and the juices run clear, 5 to 6 minutes.

Remove the patties from the pan and let rest for 3 minutes. Place one or two mushrooms on each of two, three, or four plates. Top each mushroom with a turkey burger and optional toppings and condiments of your choice.

Per serving: Protein: 23g • Calories: 283 • Dietary Fiber: 2g

Serve with unlimited salad, fruit, and nonstarchy vegetables and ½ cup grains.

Turkey Meat Loaf

Flavorful Tomato Sauce (page 287) is used in place of the usual sugar-loaded ketchup or tomato paste usually found on meat loaf. Whole Wheat Bread Crumbs (page 293) and a little Parmigiano-Reggiano add a nice texture.

Makes 4 servings

½ cup Whole Wheat Bread Crumbs (page 293)

½ teaspoon chopped fresh thyme or a heaping ⅛ teaspoon dried thyme

½ teaspoon ground black pepper

¼ teaspoon salt

2 tablespoons freshly grated Parmigiano-Reggiano

1½ pounds minced turkey

¼ cup plus 2 tablespoons Tomato Sauce (page 287)

2 large egg whites

2 teaspoons Worcestershire sauce

Chopped fresh parsley, for garnish

Preheat the oven to 350°F.

Season the bread crumbs in a medium bowl with the thyme, pepper, and salt. Add the cheese and stir well to combine.

Combine the turkey, ¼ cup of the Tomato Sauce, egg whites, and Worcestershire sauce in a large bowl and mix well with your fingers or a rubber spatula. Add the seasoned bread crumb mixture and gently mix. Transfer the meat to a 1-pound loaf pan and form into a loaf shape. Top with the remaining 2 tablespoons Tomato Sauce, spreading it evenly across the top with the back of a spoon. Bake the meat loaf until the juices run clear, 50 to 60 minutes.

Remove from the oven and let stand for 10 minutes before serving. Slice and serve hot, garnished with chopped parsley.

Per serving: Protein: 35g • Calories: 351 • Dietary Fiber: 2g

PORK

Roasted Pork Tenderloin

Two lean pork tenderloins are usually packaged together, with each weighing between 12 and 16 ounces. The recipe below is for cooking 24 ounces, or two small tenderloins. If you wish, you can double the amount of marinade. Once it's cooked, you can slice and freeze the leftover tenderloin in portions for future meals.

There are endless ways to serve pork when cooked this way. Try the Lemon-Artichoke Sauce (page 283). Roasted pork is also delicious served cold on top of a salad with some Mango Salsa (page 289) or Pico de Gallo (page 290).

Makes 4 servings

24 ounces pork tenderloin

¼ cup dry white wine or 2 tablespoons white wine or sherry vinegar

4 teaspoons Worcestershire sauce

1 tablespoon Dijon mustard

1½ teaspoons chopped garlic

1 teaspoon fresh thyme leaves or ¼ teaspoon dried thyme

½ teaspoon ground black pepper

Place the pork in a large resealable plastic bag. Whisk together the remaining ingredients in a small bowl. Pour the mixture into the bag with the pork, turning to coat evenly. Seal the bag and place inside a baking dish. Refrigerate the pork and let marinate for at least 4 and up to 6 hours.

Preheat the oven to 425°F. Remove the pork from the bag, place it inside a large baking dish, and let it come to room temperature.

Discard the marinade. Roast the pork until an instant-read thermometer inserted into the thickest part of the meat reaches an internal temperature of 155°F, 20 to 25 minutes. Remove the pork from the oven and let it rest for 5 minutes before slicing. Serve hot. (The pork can be tightly wrapped and refrigerated for up to 3 days.)

Per serving: Protein: 36g • Calories: 199 • Dietary Fiber: 0g

Serve with unlimited salad, fruit, and nonstarchy vegetables and ½ cup grains.

Pork Chops with Dijon Mustard Sauce

Boneless pork chops—more like cutlets—are a lean protein and can be ready in just minutes. Trim off all the fat before cooking.

Makes 4 servings

4 boneless center-cut rib or loin pork chops (6 ounces each)

½ teaspoon salt

1 teaspoon ground black pepper

2 teaspoons plus ½ teaspoon extra-virgin olive oil

¼ cup chopped onions

½ teaspoon crushed garlic

¼ cup dry white wine

1 teaspoon lemon juice, or to taste

¾ cup low-sodium chicken stock or vegetable stock

2 tablespoons Dijon mustard

2 teaspoons chopped tarragon or parsley

Preheat the oven to 350°F.

Season both sides of the pork with the salt and pepper.

Heat 2 teaspoons of the oil in a large nonstick skillet over medium-high heat. Add the pork to the pan and sear for 2 minutes. Turn and cook for 1 minute on the second side. Remove the pan from the heat. Transfer the pork to a baking dish and roast until cooked through, 8 to 12 minutes.

Return the pan to medium heat. Add the remaining ½ teaspoon oil and the onions and garlic to the browned bits remaining in the pan and cook, stirring with a wooden spoon, until the onions are soft, 1½ to 2 minutes. Add the wine and 1 teaspoon of the lemon juice and cook until nearly evaporated, about 30 seconds. Add the stock and stir to incorporate. Increase the heat, bring the stock to a simmer, and cook until the liquid is reduced by half, 4 to 5 minutes. Stir in the mustard and tarragon, and adjust the seasoning to taste with more lemon juice, if needed. Remove from the heat.

Place one or two pork chops on each of four large plates. Spoon the sauce over each pork chop and serve immediately.

Per serving: Protein: 35g • Calories: 288 • Dietary Fiber: 0g

Serve with unlimited salad, fruit, and nonstarchy vegetables and ½ cup grains.

FISH

Fish Fillets Baked in Foil Packets

The foil packet oven cooking method works well for fish fillets of any size. The thickness of the fillets will determine the cooking time—thin fillets (such as trout, tilapia, flounder, and striped bass) will take only 12 to 15 minutes. Meatier fish with thicker fillets, such as salmon, halibut, or grouper, will take 16 to 20 minutes.

Makes 4 servings

4 fish fillets (6 ounces each)

¼ teaspoon salt

⅛ teaspoon ground black pepper or white pepper

2 tablespoons fresh lemon juice

2 tablespoons dry white wine or water

3 tablespoons chopped spring onions, green tops only

2 tablespoons chopped fresh parsley or tarragon

Preheat the oven to 350°F. Cut 4 sheets of aluminum foil, approximately 8 x 12 inches. Lay 1 fillet in the center of each piece of foil and season lightly with the salt and pepper. Pour the lemon juice and wine around the sides and over the fillets, and sprinkle the spring onions and herbs over the tops. Draw the sides of the foil upward and around the fish, crimping to tightly seal. Place the foil packets on a baking sheet and roast until the fillets are just opaque and cooked through, 12 to 15 minutes for thin fillets, and 16 to 20 minutes for thicker ones. Place each foil packet on a plate. At the table, slice open the foil with a knife.

Per serving: Protein: 35g • Calories: 253 • Dietary Fiber: 0g

Spicy Lemon Trout Fillets

These small trout fillets will cook very quickly, making this an ideal weeknight dinner choice. You can substitute any small, firm, white fish fillets, such as flounder, sole, tilapia, or scrod. Serve any leftover trout on top of mixed greens or baby spinach for an easy lunch the next day.

If you prefer a meatier fish, use salmon, monkfish, or grouper fillets instead. Those fillets will be thicker, so the cooking time will be longer.

Makes 4 servings

1 tablespoon fresh lemon juice

2 teaspoons extra-virgin olive oil

1½ teaspoons fresh thyme leaves or ½ teaspoon dried thyme

½ teaspoon salt

½ teaspoon paprika

⅛ teaspoon cayenne, or to taste

4 trout fillets (6 ounces each)

4 lemon wedges, for garnish

Preheat the oven to 400°F. Cover a baking sheet with aluminum foil.

Whisk together the lemon juice, olive oil, thyme, salt, paprika, and cayenne in a small bowl. Spoon 2 teaspoons of the mixture evenly across the bottom of the prepared baking sheet and arrange the fillets 1 inch apart on top. Drizzle the remaining lemon juice mixture evenly over the fillets and bake until opaque and just cooked through, 5 to 7 minutes.

Remove the fish from the oven and place two small fillets or one large fillet on each of four plates. Garnish each plate with a lemon wedge and serve immediately.

Per serving: Protein: 35g • Calories: 269 • Dietary Fiber: 0g

Baked Whole Fish

This simple preparation and light sauce allow the fresh fish flavors to shine. Make this with any small, whole, firm-textured white fish, such as speckled trout, rainbow trout, bream, branzino, or bass. Once the bones, heads, and tails are removed, you'll have the right amount of protein.

Makes 4 servings

4 small whole fish (about 1–1½ pounds each), scaled and cleaned

1 teaspoon extra-virgin olive oil

2 lemons, each sliced into 6 rounds

⅓ cup finely chopped fresh parsley, divided

Salt

Ground black pepper

Preheat the oven to 400°F.

Cut three small diagonal slits into the skin on both sides of each fish, being careful not to cut through the flesh. Lightly rub each fish on both sides with the olive oil and place in a single layer on a baking sheet lined with aluminum foil. Place one lemon slice and 1 table-spoon of the parsley underneath each fish. Place one lemon slice and 1 teaspoon of the remaining parsley inside each fish cavity. Place the one remaining lemon slice on top of each fish. Lightly season the outsides and insides of the fish with salt and pepper. Bake uncovered until the flesh is opaque and cooked through but still moist, about 20 minutes, depending on the size of the fish. To serve, place one fish on each of four large plates. Serve immediately.

Per serving: Protein: 32g • Calories: 211 • Dietary Fiber: 1g

Serve with unlimited salad, fruit, and nonstarchy vegetables and ½ cup grains.

SHRIMP

Boiled Shrimp

This method of boiling also can be used to infuse flavor into those large, preboiled and frozen shrimp you find in large packages at some big-box stores. Infuse the water, as called for here; boil the defrosted shrimp for 1 to 1½ minutes; and then shock them in a bowl of ice water. If you want spicier shrimp, add more cayenne pepper and throw in a few peeled and smashed garlic cloves. Accompany the shrimp with boiled artichokes and carrots, serve with the Coleslaw (page 243) or Asian Slaw (page 242), or toss them with salad greens.

Makes 4 servings

1 small onion, quartered and peeled

½ cup chopped celery

1 lemon, quartered

2 bay leaves

2 teaspoons salt

1½ teaspoons cayenne, or to taste

1½ pounds peeled shrimp, at room temperature

Fill a large bowl with ice and water.

Place the onion, celery, lemon quarters, bay leaves, salt, and cayenne in a medium pot with 3 quarts of water and bring to the boil. Add the shrimp, bring the water back to the boil, and cook the shrimp for 4 minutes (set a kitchen timer). Drain the shrimp in a colander and immediately put them in the bowl of ice water. Drain the shrimp and serve chilled. (The boiled shrimp will keep, covered and refrigerated, for up to 3 days.)

Per serving: Protein: 35g • Calories: 210 • Dietary Fiber: 2g

EGGS

Eggs Baked in Tomato Cups

The inclusion of Ricotta Creamed Spinach makes this dish a powerhouse of nutrients! And the beautiful presentation will make this an impressive company brunch dish; double the recipe for a large crowd.

Makes 4 servings

4 large ripe tomatoes (about 8 ounces each)

¼ cup Ricotta Creamed Spinach (page 251)

4 large eggs

¼ teaspoon salt

⅛ teaspoon freshly ground black pepper

2 tablespoons freshly grated Parmigiano-Reggiano or low-fat mozzarella

Chopped fresh parsley, for garnish (optional)

Preheat the oven to 400°F.

Slice the top quarter from each tomato and remove the seeds and pulp, leaving a hollow shell. Place the tomatoes in a 9 x 9-inch baking dish or in individual ½-cup ramekins.

Spoon 1 tablespoon of the spinach into the bottom of each tomato and break 1 egg into each on top of the spinach. Season the eggs lightly with the salt and pepper. Bake until the eggs are set and the tomatoes are soft, 21 to 23 minutes for soft yolks and 24 to 27 minutes for hard yolks. (The eggs will continue to cook in the tomatoes once they are removed from the oven.) Sprinkle 1½ teaspoons of the cheese over the top of each egg and garnish, if desired, with the parsley. Serve immediately.

Per serving: Protein: 11g • Calories: 141 • Dietary Fiber: 2g

Berry-Spinach Frittata

This one-person dish is packed with 3 ounces of protein from the eggs, making it a smart choice for a light lunch or supper. Top it with Orange-Mint Yogurt Sauce (page 284) for added protein and flavor. And perhaps best of all, this frittata can be made with fresh or frozen berries, straight from the freezer. Substitute any other fresh or frozen fruit, but make sure that it is cut into uniform pieces.

Makes 1 serving

2 large egg whites

1 large egg

Pinch of salt

Pinch of ground black pepper

½ teaspoon extra-virgin olive oil

½ cup fresh or frozen strawberries, cut into ½-inch pieces

½ cup fresh or frozen blueberries

½ cup finely chopped fresh or frozen spinach

½ teaspoon finely grated orange zest

¼ cup Orange-Mint Yogurt Sauce (page 284)

Preheat the oven to 375°F.

Beat together the egg whites, whole egg, salt, and pepper in a small bowl and set aside.

Heat the oil in a small nonstick ovenproof skillet over medium heat, swirling the pan to coat the bottom and sides. Add the strawberries, blueberries, and spinach and cook, stirring, for 1½ minutes if frozen or 30 to 45 seconds if fresh. Add the zest and stir. Add the eggs. Tilting the pan and using a rubber spatula, push the eggs around the berries and spinach, allowing the uncooked eggs to run to the center of the pan, about 15 seconds. Let the eggs cook undisturbed until they start to just set around the edge, about 1 minute.

Place the pan in the oven and bake until the eggs are cooked through, about 12 minutes.

Remove the pan from the oven. Using a rubber spatula, slide the frittata out onto a large plate. Spoon the yogurt sauce over the eggs and serve immediately.

Per serving: Protein: 18g • Calories: 224 • Dietary Fiber: 4g

Serve with unlimited salad, fruit, and nonstarchy vegetables and ½ cup grains.

Courgette Torte

Lightly golden and puffy, this oven-baked torte can be enjoyed for lunch or dinner.

Makes 6 servings

Vegetable oil spray

1½ teaspoons extra-virgin olive oil

½ cup chopped onions

1½ teaspoons crushed garlic

1¼ pounds fresh courgettes, ends trimmed and grated (about 4 cups)

½ teaspoon salt

¼ teaspoon ground black pepper

Pinch of cayenne (optional)

1 tablespoon chopped fresh basil or 1 teaspoon dried basil

2 teaspoons chopped fresh parsley or ¾ teaspoon dried parsley

2 large egg whites

1 large egg

½ cup plus 1 tablespoon Whole Wheat Bread Crumbs (page 293)

¼ cup plus 1 tablespoon shredded fat-free mozzarella cheese

¼ cup grated Parmigiano-Reggiano

Preheat the oven to 350°F. Spray an 8-inch round baking dish with vegetable oil spray and set aside. (Alternatively, you can use an 8 x 8-inch square dish.)

Heat the oil in a large, heavy nonstick skillet over medium heat. Add the onions and cook, stirring, until soft, 3½ to 4 minutes. Add the garlic and cook, stirring, until fragrant, 30 to 45 seconds. Add the courgette and cook, stirring, until it gives off its liquid and is wilted, but is still bright green and not completely dry, 5 to 6 minutes. Add the salt, pepper, cayenne (if using), basil, and parsley, and cook, stirring, until incorporated, 20 seconds. Remove the pan from the heat and let the mixture cool, stirring occasionally, about 6 minutes.

Beat the egg whites and egg together in a large bowl. Add the cooled courgette mixture and stir rapidly to combine. Add the remaining ingredients and stir to combine. (The mixture will be slightly wet.) Pour into the prepared baking dish and bake until the torte is set, risen, and lightly golden, about 35 minutes. Remove from the oven and let cool for 5 minutes before serving.

Per serving: Protein: 17g • Calories: 216 • Dietary Fiber: 4g

Serve with unlimited salad, fruit, and nonstarchy vegetables and ½ cup grains.

TOFU

Oven-Roasted Tofu on Baby Spinach

Tofu readily takes on the flavors of whatever it's marinated in. This marinade has traditional Asian flavors—citrus, soy, ginger, garlic, and toasted sesame oil. Once it's cooked, serve it on a bed of baby spinach leaves accompanied by Brown Rice (page 258).

Makes 4 servings

2 (14-ounce) packages firm tofu, drained

¼ cup fresh lime juice

2 tablespoons fresh orange juice

3 tablespoons low-sodium soy sauce

2 tablespoons peeled and chopped fresh ginger

4 teaspoons chopped garlic

1 tablespoon toasted sesame oil

1 teaspoon finely grated orange zest

½ teaspoon red pepper flakes

Baby spinach, for serving

Dijon Mustard Lemon Dressing (page 281)

Sliced spring onions, for garnish

Line a baking dish with paper towels. Halve the tofu crosswise and cut it into ½-inch-thick slices. Place on the paper towels and top with a layer of several paper towels. Place another baking dish (or a skillet) on top and weight with a heavy can. Let sit until well drained, 10 to 15 minutes.

To make the marinade, combine the lime juice, orange juice, soy sauce, ginger, garlic, sesame oil, orange zest, and red pepper flakes in a small bowl. Remove the dish, weight, and paper towels from the baking dish and place the tofu flat in the baking dish. Pour the marinade ingredients over the tofu, cover, and refrigerate for at least 1 and up to 4 hours.

Preheat the oven to 375°F and let the tofu and its marinade come to room temperature. Bake, turning once, until the tofu is firm and golden brown, about 30 minutes. Remove from the oven and let cool slightly. Place the greens in a large bowl and toss lightly with 2 teaspoons to 2 tablespoons of the dressing, depending on the number of portions. Arrange the greens on four large plates, and place the tofu on top. Garnish each portion with sliced spring onions and serve.

Per serving: Protein: 16g • Calories: 221 • Dietary Fiber: 1g

Serve with unlimited salad, fruit, and nonstarchy vegetables and ½ cup grains.

SALADS AND VEGETABLES

Meet your new BFFs. Salads and vegetables will be your new sidekicks—the whole foods you can count on to deliver the nutrients you need without compromising that waistline you've been dreaming of. Even when you think you've made the last salad recipe on earth or sautéed more vegetables than you can count, you really haven't! Salads and veggies are going to be a huge part of your diet, and they'll never fail to deliver on energy, taste, and filling satisfaction.

The Age-Defying Diet offers a huge range of health-promoting, antioxidant-rich salads and vegetables that you can eat at every whole-food meal. Stock up on your favorites once or twice a week, and wash and prepare them as soon as you get home from the market. That way there will always be some of your favorites to nibble on, since fruits and nonstarchy vegetables are a bottomless delight on the Age-Defying Diet. Be sure to keep a variety of salad greens ready to mix and match and top with other vegetables. A quick salad can fill you up and is easy to tote on the go!

Asian Slaw

This recipe is made using half of a 14-ounce bag. But it doubles easily if you wish to take it to work the next day, or to serve a large group.

Makes 3 cups, or 4 servings

1 tablespoon fresh lime juice

1 tablespoon rice wine vinegar

1 tablespoon chopped fresh coriander

1 tablespoon chopped fresh mint

1½ teaspoons soy sauce

1½ teaspoons chopped fresh ginger

1 teaspoon toasted sesame oil

¼ teaspoon sriracha or chili paste

¼ teaspoon salt

7 ounces packaged coleslaw mix

2 tablespoons thinly sliced spring onions, green tops only

1 teaspoon chopped unsalted roasted peanuts

To make the dressing, combine the lime juice, vinegar, coriander, mint, soy sauce, ginger, sesame oil, sriracha, and salt in a bowl and whisk to combine.

Place the coleslaw mix, spring onions, and peanuts in a large bowl. Add the dressing and stir well to coat evenly. Cover and refrigerate for at least 1 and up to 8 hours before serving. (The slaw will keep, covered and refrigerated, for up to 4 days.)

Per serving: Protein: 1g • Calories: 32 • Dietary Fiber: 1g

Coleslaw

Instead of using high-calorie mayonnaise or sour cream for the dressing, this recipe calls for my nonfat-yogurt-based Mayonnaise (page 282). It can be doubled easily. If you like, add some grated apple to the mix.

Makes 3 cups, or 4 servings

7 ounces packaged coleslaw mix

6 tablespoons Mayonnaise (page 282)

¼ cup sliced spring onions, green tops only

2 tablespoons chopped fresh parsley

½ teaspoon salt

¼ teaspoon ground black pepper

Combine all the ingredients in a large bowl and stir well to coat evenly. Cover and refrigerate for at least 1 and up to 8 hours before serving. (The slaw will keep, covered and refrigerated, for up to 4 days.)

Per serving: Protein: 3g • Calories: 39 • Dietary Fiber: 1g

Waldorf Salad

The secret to this salad is to chop the apples, celery, and grapes into pieces of the same size—about ½ inch each. Tossing the chopped apples with lemon juice first prevents them from browning. You can serve this as an unlimited salad or snack, but don't increase the amount of nuts.

Makes 2 cups, or 4 servings

1 apple, such as Gala or Fuji, cored and chopped

2 teaspoons fresh lemon juice

½ cup chopped celery

½ cup quartered red seedless grapes

3 tablespoons Mayonnaise (page 282)

4 teaspoons chopped toasted walnuts or pecans

1 tablespoon chopped fresh parsley

2 teaspoons chopped spring onions

¾ teaspoon finely grated lemon zest

¼ teaspoon ground black pepper

⅛ teaspoon salt

Toss the apples and lemon juice in a medium bowl. Add the remaining ingredients and mix well. Serve immediately, or cover tightly and refrigerate until ready to serve. (The salad will keep, covered and refrigerated, for up to 3 days.)

Per serving: Protein: 1g • Calories: 87 • Dietary Fiber: 1g

Waldorf Chicken/Turkey Salad: For a main course, add chopped-up pieces of Chicken Breasts Baked in Foil Packets (page 215), Pan-Cooked Chicken Breasts (page 216), or Roasted Turkey Breast (page 222).

Boiled or Steamed Vegetables

The secret to delicious vegetables that retain the maximum amount of nutrients is to cook them just until they are tender and retain a slight crunch. You can do this either by quickly cooking them in boiling water on top of the stove, or by steaming them in the microwave. Both methods are given below, and both methods also work for frozen vegetables.

Cooking times depend on the type of vegetable and how it is cut up. A squeeze of fresh lemon or orange juice and a teaspoon of extra-virgin olive oil with a dash of salt and pepper are all you need to enjoy quickly cooked fresh or frozen vegetables. Any leftover cooked vegetables can be refrigerated and served cold in salads or smoothies.

Makes 6 servings

1 small head broccoli, trimmed and cut into florets

1 small head cauliflower, cored and cut into florets

½ pound carrots, ends trimmed, peeled, and sliced into rounds

½ pound fresh green beans, trimmed and strings removed

½ pound mangetout

½ pound medium courgette, sliced into ¼-inch rounds

½ pound butternut squash, sliced into ¼-inch rounds

Bring a pot of lightly salted water to the boil. Add the vegetables, return to a low boil, and cook uncovered until just tender, 3 to 6 minutes. Drain in a colander and season lightly to taste. Serve immediately.

Alternatively, place the vegetables in a microwaveable baking dish large enough to hold them in a single layer. Add 1 tablespoon of water, cover tightly with plastic wrap, and microwave on high until just tender, 2½ to 5 minutes, depending upon the power of the oven.

Per serving: Protein: 6g • Calories: 75 • Dietary Fiber: 5g

Roasted Vegetables

Roasting vegetables brings out their inherent sweetness. The vegetables listed below are just a jumping-off point. Cook any fresh vegetables using this basic technique, keeping in mind that cooking times will vary depending upon the vegetable used and how it is cut.

The key to roasting vegetables successfully is to cut all pieces the same size and not overcrowd them on the baking sheet; crowding will cause them to steam.

For a delicious side dish, cube the vegetables instead of slicing them into sticks before roasting, and toss them with pasta, brown rice, or any other cooked grain.

Makes 6 servings

½ pound asparagus, trimmed

½ pound brussels sprouts

3 medium carrots, quartered lengthwise and crosswise into
    4 equal sticks

3 medium parsnips, quartered lengthwise and crosswise into
    4 equal sticks

3 medium courgettes, or butternut squash, quartered lengthwise
    and crosswise into 4 equal sticks

1 red onion, cut into wedges

1 tablespoon extra-virgin olive oil

½ teaspoon salt

¼ teaspoon ground black pepper

Chopped fresh herbs (optional)

Preheat the oven to 425°F. Cover a baking sheet with aluminum foil.

Place the vegetables on the baking sheet and toss with the oil, salt, and pepper to coat. Roast until tender and slightly caramelized, 20 to 40 minutes, depending upon the vegetable, shaking the pan once or twice if necessary for the vegetables to cook evenly. Serve hot or at room temperature as a side dish or topping for grains, tossing with chopped fresh herbs of your choice before serving, if desired.

Per serving: Protein: 4g • Calories: 107 • Dietary Fiber: 7g

Cooked Greens

Mustard greens, kale, chard, spring greens, and turnip greens are cruciferous vegetables from the same family as broccoli and cabbage. They are absolutely packed with good-for-you nutrients. Kale and spring greens are a bit more bitter, while mustard and turnip greens are slightly peppery. The orange juice is used in place of the usual sugar or cane syrup to balance the bitterness of the greens. Use more or less to suit your tastes. Spring greens and mustard greens are tougher and take longer to cook, and you may need to add more stock during the cooking time if they get too dry.

Makes 4 servings

2 teaspoons extra-virgin olive oil

½ cup chopped onions

1 teaspoon crushed garlic

½ teaspoon salt

¼ teaspoon ground black pepper

¼ teaspoon red pepper flakes

2 bunches (about 2 pounds) fresh greens, washed well, tough stems (and spring green ribs) removed, and torn into pieces; or 1 pound frozen chopped greens, thawed

1–2 tablespoons fresh orange juice, to taste

1 tablespoon red wine vinegar

½–1 cup vegetable stock or water, or more as needed

Hot sauce (optional)

Heat the oil in a large nonstick skillet over medium heat. Add the onions and cook, stirring, until soft and starting to turn golden brown, about 5 minutes. Add the garlic, salt, black pepper, and red pepper flakes and cook, stirring, until fragrant, 30 seconds. Add the greens in batches, turning them and adding more as they begin to wilt. Add the orange juice and vinegar and stir well. Add ½ cup of the vegetable stock and bring to a simmer. Cook, stirring occasionally, until the greens are wilted and tender, 15 to 30 minutes, adding more stock as needed for a longer cooking time. Serve hot with hot sauce on the side.

Per serving: Protein: 5g • Calories: 98 • Dietary Fiber: 8g

Sautéed Spinach with Garlic

Quickly tossed in a hot skillet, sautéed spinach with garlic goes with just about anything you can think of—whether meat, fish, fowl, tofu, or eggs.

Makes 4 servings

2 teaspoons extra-virgin olive oil

2 teaspoons crushed garlic

1 pound fresh baby spinach, washed

1 teaspoon fresh lemon juice or orange juice

⅛ teaspoon salt

⅛ teaspoon ground black pepper

Heat the oil in a large nonstick skillet over medium-high heat. Add the garlic and cook, stirring, until fragrant, 45 seconds to 1 minute. Add one-third of the spinach and cook, stirring, until it is almost wilted, 1 to 2 minutes. Add the remaining spinach in two batches, and up to 2 teaspoons of water as necessary to keep it from sticking to the pan; cook, stirring, until all the spinach is wilted, about 4 minutes. Add the lemon juice, salt, and pepper and stir to combine before serving.

Per serving: Protein: 3g • Calories: 48 • Dietary Fiber: 2g

Ricotta Creamed Spinach

This low-calorie creamed spinach recipe couldn't be easier to make since it calls for frozen chopped spinach. It can be used as a stuffing for the Roasted Pork Tenderloin (page 226) and the Stuffed Chicken Breasts (page 217), or incorporated into egg dishes (Eggs Baked in Tomato Cups, page 234), as well as served as a side vegetable.

Buy frozen chopped spinach in the larger bags in bulk to keep on hand for this dish, soups, or smoothies. Note that 1 cup of frozen spinach cooked in the microwave, as done here, will yield about ¼ cup when squeezed dry. This recipe can easily be doubled.

Makes 4 servings

5 cups frozen chopped spinach

2 teaspoons extra-virgin olive oil

5 tablespoons chopped onions

6 tablespoons half-fat ricotta cheese

5 teaspoons fresh lemon juice

½ teaspoon salt

¼ teaspoon ground black pepper

¼ teaspoon freshly grated nutmeg (optional)

Place the spinach in a large microwaveable bowl with 3 tablespoons of water. Cover tightly with plastic wrap and microwave on high until cooked through and tender, 5 to 6 minutes. Let sit covered for 1 minute.

Remove from the microwave. Transfer to a fine-mesh strainer, pressing down on the spinach with the back of a heavy spoon to expel all excess liquid.

Heat the oil in a large nonstick skillet over medium-high heat. Add the onions and cook, stirring, until soft, about 3 minutes. Add the spinach and cook, stirring, until dry, 30 seconds to 1 minute. Add the ricotta, lemon juice, salt, pepper, and nutmeg (if using); stir well to combine, and cook until hot, 1 to 2 minutes. Serve immediately.

Per serving: Protein: 4g • Calories: 68 • Dietary Fiber: 1g

Steamed Baby Pak Choi

This little member of the cabbage family also goes by the name Chinese cabbage, and translated from the Cantonese means "white vegetable." It's tender, sweet, and delicious on its own or as a side dish. Cooking pak choi in stock adds a boost of extra flavor, but using water is fine.

Makes 4 servings

1½ cups low-sodium chicken stock or water

1 pound baby pak choi, trimmed and cut in half lengthwise

½ teaspoon toasted sesame oil

¼ teaspoon soy sauce

Pinch of red pepper flakes

2 teaspoons chopped unsalted roasted peanuts

Place the stock and pak choi in a large skillet and bring to a simmer over medium-high heat. Cook, turning occasionally, until the pak choi is tender, 10 to 12 minutes. Transfer the pak choi with tongs to a bowl. Transfer ¼ cup of the stock from the pan to a bowl. Stir in the sesame oil, soy sauce, and pepper flakes. Pour the sauce over the pak choi, top with the peanuts, and serve.

Per serving: Protein: 3g • Calories: 34 • Dietary Fiber: 1g

Roasted Aubergine

You'll have many uses for this aubergine. Serve the aubergine as a whole-grain topping, as a dip with endive leaves, or as a side dish with lemon juice and parsley.

Makes 1–1½ cups; 2 tablespoons per serving

1 (1-pound) aubergine, unpeeled, cut in half lengthwise

½ teaspoon salt

½ teaspoon ground black pepper

Lemon wedges (optional)

Chopped fresh parsley (optional)

Preheat the oven to 400°F. Line a baking sheet with aluminum foil. Season the aubergine halves with salt and pepper. Place them, cut side down, on the prepared baking sheet and roast until the skin is wrinkled and the flesh is very soft, 50 minutes to 1 hour.

Remove the halves from the oven and let them rest on the baking sheet until cool enough to handle, 15 to 20 minutes. Using two forks, shred the aubergine; discard the skin before serving.

Per serving: Protein: 1g • Calories: 20 • Dietary Fiber: 3g

Roasted Peppers

Roasting red, yellow, or orange peppers intensifies their flavors. Here are three easy ways to roast peppers—choose the method most suitable for you. Roasted peppers can be used with fish, chicken, or salads. Feel free to double the recipe.

Makes about 1 cup; 2 tablespoons per serving

2 large red peppers

2 large yellow peppers

Method 1: Preheat a grill to medium-high heat. Place the peppers on the grill and roast, turning with tongs, until the peppers are charred black on all sides, 5 to 10 minutes.

Method 2: Roast the peppers over a gas burner. Preheat a stovetop burner to medium-high heat. Set the peppers one at a time onto the burner's metal grate and cook, turning, until charred on all sides, 5 to 10 minutes.

Method 3: Cook the peppers in the oven. Place the oven rack at its highest setting and preheat the grill to high. Put the peppers on a baking sheet covered with aluminum foil. Grill the peppers, turning, until charred on all sides, 5 to 10 minutes.

Set the roasted peppers in a large bowl. Cover with plastic wrap and let steam for 10 minutes. Uncover and let sit until cool enough to handle. Working over the sink, peel the charred skin from the peppers and remove the stems and seeds. Roughly chop and use as directed, or store refrigerated in an airtight container. (The peppers will keep refrigerated for up to 3 days.)

Per serving: Protein: 2g • Calories: 48 • Dietary Fiber: 4g

Courgette Noodles

Who says you can't eat noodles? These vegetable ribbons make a great substitution for pasta. If there's no Pesto (page 286) on hand, then toss the "noodles" with a little grated lemon zest and chopped fresh basil, mint, and parsley, or some Tomato Sauce (page 287). You can use this basic pan-cooking method for cucumber and carrot ribbons as well. Just adjust the cooking time accordingly.

Makes 4 servings

2 medium courgettes or butternut squash (7–8 ounces each), ends trimmed and halved lengthwise

1 teaspoon extra-virgin olive oil

1½ teaspoons chopped garlic

Pinch of salt

Pinch of freshly ground black pepper

2 tablespoons vegetable stock or water

2 tablespoons Pesto (page 286)

Lay one courgette half on its side on a chopping board, grasping the end between your index finger and thumb, cut side out. Run a vegetable peeler in a single motion down the top length of the courgette to make a long ribbon. Repeat, turning the courgette over halfway through, on the other side. Repeat with the remaining courgette. (You will have 4 to 5 cups of ribbons.)

Heat a large nonstick skillet over medium heat. Add the oil and when it's hot, add the garlic, salt, and pepper. Cook, stirring, until the garlic is fragrant, 20 to 30 seconds. Add the courgette to the pan, toss with a spatula, and cook undisturbed for 1 minute. Toss the courgette again to redistribute the bottom noodles to the top, add the stock, and increase the heat to high. Let cook undisturbed until the noodles are wilted and tender, 1½ to 3 minutes. Stir and remove from the heat. Toss the noodles with the Pesto. Serve immediately.

Per serving: Protein: 1g • Calories: 47 • Dietary Fiber: 0g

GRAINS

Grains. They've got a bad reputation thanks to fad diets that claim all carbohydrates are bad for you. Nothing could be further from the truth. Never-processed whole grains are not only tasty and filling, but also good-for-you sources of fiber, antioxidants, vitamins, and minerals. *Refined* grains, such as white rice and the white flour found in regular pasta, breakfast cereals, and snack foods, are to be avoided because all of their nutritional value has been stripped away during processing.

Whole grains contain 100 percent of the grain kernel, including the bran, germ, and endosperm with all their nutritional power. The secret is to eat just a small amount to obtain their satisfying nourishment. The best part? Grains are filling thanks to all that mighty fiber, and when you're full and satiated, you don't have room to eat any of the junk that used to fill up your daily diet. So throw away your old notions about grains, and try these tips for simmering up some of the tasty whole kind.

• Cook a full batch of each grain, and then divide into ½-cup serving sizes and refrigerate or freeze.

• No time to cook your grains? Purchase a container of steamed brown rice from your local Chinese restaurant, or cooked quinoa from a salad bar, or frozen grains from your grocer's freezer. Divide into ½-cup servings. Refrigerate or freeze any leftovers for future meals.

Amaranth

While it's often called a grain, amaranth is actually the seed of a plant that has been cultivated for thousands of years and was a dietary staple of the pre-Columbus Aztecs. It is high in protein, iron, and lysine, an essential amino acid.

Cooked amaranth has a sweet, slightly nutty flavor, and like other grains it's delicious with ground cinnamon, fresh berries, and toasted nuts added to it. Be careful not to overcook amaranth or it will become mushy and unappetizing.

Makes 6 servings

1 cup amaranth seeds

2½ cups water

Combine the amaranth and water in a pot and bring to the boil. Reduce the heat to low, cover, and simmer until all the water is absorbed and the grains are tender, 18 to 20 minutes. Remove the pan from the heat, uncover, and let rest for 5 minutes. Fluff the amaranth with a fork and serve immediately.

Per serving: Protein: 2g • Calories: 42 • Dietary Fiber: 1g

Brown Rice

Makes 6 servings

2¼ cups water

½ teaspoon salt

1 cup long-grain brown rice

Bring the water and salt to the boil in a medium pot. Add the rice, stir, cover, and reduce the heat to low. Simmer, covered and undisturbed, until the water is absorbed and the rice is tender, 40 to 50 minutes. Remove from the heat, uncover, and let rest for 5 minutes. Fluff the rice with a fork and serve immediately.

Per serving: Protein: 2g • Calories: 114 • Dietary Fiber: 1g

Bulgur

Bulgur wheat is cracked wheat that has been parboiled before packaging to shorten its cooking time. It is made in a variety of grinds, from extra-fine to coarse, with fine and medium grind the most common; the finer the grind, the faster it cooks (or steeps). As with most grains, you can use a simple ratio of 2 parts water to 1 part bulgur should you wish to cook a larger portion. And also as with other grains, bulgur often is used in place of rice and in salads and can be flavored in a variety of ways.

Makes 6 servings

1 cup bulgur wheat

⅛ teaspoon salt

Place the bulgur wheat and salt in a large bowl. Bring 2 cups of water to the boil. Pour the water over the bulgur, cover, and let stand until the water is absorbed and the grains are plump, 10 to 20 minutes. Drain in a strainer as needed to get rid of extra water and return to the bowl. Fluff the bulgur with a fork and let stand for 5 minutes. Eat hot or at room temperature, or cover and chill to serve in salads. (Bulgur will keep, tightly covered, in the refrigerator for up to 5 days.)

Per serving: Protein: 3g • Calories: 80 • Dietary Fiber: 4g

Couscous

Couscous can be served with meat, chicken, fish, shrimp, or vegetables. I stir in a little fresh orange zest and parsley along with a splash of orange juice to the couscous once it is cooked.

Makes 6 servings

1 cup couscous

⅛ teaspoon salt

Place the couscous and salt in a large bowl. Bring 2 cups of water to the boil. Pour the water over the couscous, cover, and let stand until the water is absorbed and the grains are plump, 10 to 20 minutes. Fluff the couscous with a fork and let stand for 5 minutes. Eat hot or at room temperature, or cover and chill to serve in salads. (Couscous will keep, tightly covered, in the refrigerator for up to 5 days.)

Per serving: Protein: 4g • Calories: 108 • Dietary Fiber: 1g

Quinoa

Quinoa has a natural resin coating that needs to be removed before cooking by rinsing or toasting. If you choose to rinse first, dry the grains in the pan for 1 minute before adding the liquid to cook them.

Makes 6 servings

1 cup quinoa

2 cups water or vegetable stock

¼ teaspoon salt

Place the quinoa in a fine-mesh strainer and rinse under cold running water until the water runs clear, about 2 minutes. Transfer the quinoa to a medium saucepan and lightly toast it over medium-low heat until any water clinging to the grains is evaporated. Add the water and salt and bring to the boil. Reduce the heat to low, cover, and simmer until tender, 12 to 15 minutes.

Alternatively, instead of rinsing, place the uncooked quinoa in a large skillet over medium heat. Toast the grains until lightly golden brown and fragrant, 2 to 3 minutes. Remove the pan from the heat and transfer the grains to a medium saucepan. Cook with the water, as above, until tender, 10 to 12 minutes.

Per serving: Protein: 4g • Calories: 108 • Dietary Fiber: 2g

Tabbouleh

Tabbouleh is traditionally made with a small amount of bulgur and large handfuls of parsley and mint and chopped cucumber and tomatoes, which makes it ideal for the Age-Defying Diet. Use this recipe as a departure point for creating your own new favorite bulgur wheat salad. For instance, you might try fresh berries or fresh or frozen peach slices or mango cubes, with fresh mint, served as an accompaniment to Boiled Shrimp (page 233).

Makes 6 servings

1 cup bulgur wheat
2 tablespoons extra-virgin olive oil
2 tablespoons fresh lemon juice
½ teaspoon salt
¼ teaspoon ground black pepper
1 cup chopped fresh parsley
⅓ cup finely sliced spring onions, green tops only
¼ cup chopped fresh mint
⅓ cup peeled, seeded, and chopped cucumber
⅓ cup seeded and chopped tomatoes

Place the bulgur wheat in a large bowl. Bring 2 cups of water to the boil. Pour the water over the bulgur, cover, and let stand until the water is absorbed and the grains are plump, 10 to 20 minutes. Drain in a strainer as needed to get rid of extra water and return to the bowl. Fluff the bulgur with a fork and let stand for 5 minutes.

Whisk together the olive oil, lemon juice, salt, and pepper in a small bowl. Add the parsley, spring onions, and mint and whisk to combine. Add the oil mixture to the bulgur wheat and toss lightly to coat the grains. Add the cucumber and tomatoes, folding to evenly distribute through the salad. Serve at room temperature, or cover and chill until ready to serve. (Tabbouleh will keep, covered, in the refrigerator for 3 days.)

Per serving: Protein: 3g • Calories: 128 • Dietary Fiber: 5g

Whole Wheat Pasta

While whole wheat pasta is packed with fiber, it still has carbohydrates. Know that different shapes and sizes of pasta will yield different amounts. Be sure to measure your portions before serving in order to stick to the recommended amount. Also be sure to buy 100% whole wheat pasta. For variety, toss the pasta with Roasted Garlic (page 292) and chopped fresh herbs, Pesto (page 286), or Tomato Sauce (page 287).

Makes 6–8 servings

6–8 ounces whole wheat pasta

1 tablespoon chicken or vegetable stock

2 teaspoons extra-virgin olive oil

¼ teaspoon salt

Bring a pot of salted water to the boil. Add the pasta, return to the boil, and cook uncovered until al dente, 7 to 10 minutes, depending upon the pasta's size and shape. Drain in a colander set in the sink and return to the pot. Add the remaining ingredients and toss to coat the pasta. Place over medium heat until hot. Serve immediately. (Leftover pasta can be kept, tightly covered and refrigerated, for up to 4 days.)

Per serving: Protein: 5g • Calories: 130 • Dietary Fiber: 3g

DESSERTS

Even doctors like me, who specialize in nutrition and weight loss, want a satisfying sweet finish to our meals every once in a while. There are times when an ice pop or a fat-free pudding just doesn't do the trick. Believe me, I know how it is. With my own sweet tooth in mind, here are some easy-to-make cookies, pies, puddings, and cakes to enjoy with your dinnertime whole meal. Again, I've done all the calorie counting and math for you; these desserts are all well within the boundaries of what you can eat on the Age-Defying Diet. The recipes make enough servings so you can share them with your family or freeze them in individual portions for future use. These desserts are easy to make. I like to make everything as easy as possible for my patients and my readers, so I have additional dessert recipes and alternative ready-made desserts on my website DrApovian.com.

Blueberry Pie Cups

These individual "pies" can be made ahead and served to your family or at the end of an elegant dinner party.

Makes 8 servings

1½ cups low-fat/lower-sugar granola

2 tablespoons orange marmalade all-fruit spread

1 pint fresh blueberries

¼ cup blueberry all-fruit spread

Preheat the oven to 350°F. Line eight muffin cups with foil liners.

In a food processor or blender, pulse the granola until it's finely chopped but with flakes of oats still present. Add the marmalade and pulse until combined. Press rounded tablespoons into the muffin cups. In a medium bowl, combine the blueberries and blueberry fruit spread, stirring until the berries are coated. Spoon into the muffin cups. Bake for 20 minutes or until the berries soften and the filling is about level with the edge of the foil liners. Cool on a wire rack. Chill before serving.

Per serving: Protein: 2g • Calories: 130 • Dietary Fiber: 3g

Cherry Fro-Yo

When you want a chilled, refreshing dessert, this cherry frozen yogurt comes together in minutes. If you prefer your fro-yo colder, put it into the freezer for a few hours.

Makes 6 servings

1 (5.3-ounce) container nonfat vanilla Greek yogurt

½–¾ cup nonfat milk

1 (12-ounce) package unsweetened frozen dark sweet cherries

¾ cup fat-free frozen whipped topping, thawed

Combine the yogurt, ½ cup of the milk, and the cherries in a blender. Blend, adding additional milk as necessary, until the mixture is smooth. Pour the mixture into a medium bowl and fold in the whipped topping. Serve immediately—or for a firmer texture, freeze for 2 to 3 hours. Freeze leftovers in an airtight container, removing from the freezer 15 to 20 minutes before serving to soften.

Per serving: Protein: 4g • Calories: 75 • Dietary Fiber: 2g

Individual Peach Cobblers

A sweetened yogurt-and-oatmeal filling is spooned into fresh peach halves and then baked until the peaches are tender. Feel free to substitute apricots or plums.

Makes 4 servings

Nonstick cooking spray

4 medium fresh peaches, halved and pitted

½ cup quick-cooking oatmeal

¼ cup nonfat vanilla Greek yogurt

3 packets Truvia or Splenda sugar substitute (each equivalent to 2 teaspoons sugar)

¼ teaspoon ground cinnamon, plus additional for dusting

Preheat the oven to 350°F. Spray an 11 x 7-inch baking pan with nonstick cooking spray. Place the peach halves, cut side up, in the baking pan. In a small bowl, combine the oats, yogurt, sweetener, and ¼ teaspoon cinnamon; stir to combine. Spoon evenly into the peach halves; sprinkle with additional cinnamon. Bake for 15 minutes or until the topping begins to turn golden and the peaches are tender. Serve while warm.

Per serving: Protein: 4g • Calories: 110 • Dietary Fiber: 4g

Chocolate Crisps

If you like, sprinkle ½ cup mini chocolate chips, unsweetened coconut, or chopped nuts over the cookies.

Makes 16 servings

⅔ cup white whole wheat flour

½ cup Stevia Extract in the Raw

2 tablespoons unsweetened cocoa powder

2 large egg whites

3 tablespoons water

4½ teaspoons vegetable oil

Mini chocolate chips, shredded unsweetened coconut, or chopped nuts (optional)

Preheat the oven to 350°F. Line two baking sheets with parchment paper.

Combine the flour, sweetener, and cocoa in a bowl; mix thoroughly. Add the egg whites, water, and oil, and stir until smooth. Spoon 1 tablespoon of the batter onto the parchment paper and spread with a spatula to a 3 x 5-inch oval. You should not be able to see through to the parchment. Repeat with the remaining batter. Six crisps will fit on each baking sheet. Crisps do not spread. Sprinkle with chips, coconut, or nuts, if you like.

Bake for 13 to 17 minutes, watching carefully the last few minutes so they do not burn. Remove from the oven and cool on the pan for 5 minutes before cooling completely on a wire rack. The cookies will continue to become crisp as they cool.

Per serving: Protein: 1g • Calories: 35 • Dietary Fiber: 1g

Pecan-Flax Crookers

You can purchase pecan meal at health food stores, or process ⅔ cup whole pecans in a food processor to make ⅔ cup pecan meal.

Makes 6 (5-cracker) servings

⅔ cup lightly packed pecan meal (finely ground pecans)

⅓ cup golden flaxseed meal (ground flaxseeds)

⅓ cup Stevia Extract in the Raw

1½ teaspoons ground cinnamon

1 large egg white

Preheat the oven to 350°F.

Combine the pecan meal, flax meal, sweetener, and cinnamon in a bowl; mix thoroughly. Add the egg white and stir until the mixture starts to form a ball. Place the dough on a sheet of parchment and top with a sheet of waxed paper (or parchment). Roll to a 9 x 10-inch rectangle. Remove the waxed paper and, using a knife, score into 1½-inch squares, leaving the squares attached.

Place the parchment paper with the squares on a baking sheet. Bake for 16 to 20 minutes, or until the crookers are deep brown but not burned. Remove the pan, and when cool enough to handle, break the crookers into squares. If necessary, turn the crookers that were in the center of the pan over and bake for an additional 2 to 3 minutes to become crisp. When they're cool, store in an airtight container.

Per serving (5 crackers): Protein: 3g • Calories: 134 • Dietary Fiber: 3g

No-Bake Kiwi Cookies

Store-bought cookies are dressed up and topped with thin slices of kiwi and a dollop of sweetened, creamy cottage cheese. Nothing could be easier.

Makes 6 servings

½ cup low-fat (2%) cottage cheese

2 packets Truvia or Splenda sugar substitute (each equivalent to 2 teaspoons sugar)

½ teaspoon lemon juice

1 kiwi, peeled

12 thin cookies

Combine the cottage cheese, sweetener, and lemon juice in a food processor. Blend until smooth.

Thinly slice the kiwi and cut the slices into quarters. Just before serving, place a small dollop (about 1 teaspoon) of the cottage cheese mixture on the center of each cookie; top with a piece of kiwi. Serve immediately.

Per serving: Protein: 3g • Calories: 70 • Dietary Fiber: 1g

Peanut-Butter-and-Chocolate-Drizzled Bananas

Salty peanut butter and sweet chocolate chips are combined and then drizzled over bananas.

Makes 4 servings

3 medium bananas, peeled and diagonally sliced

2 tablespoons reduced-fat creamy peanut butter

¼ cup water

¼ teaspoon vanilla extract

2 teaspoons mini chocolate chips

Divide the banana slices among four plates. In a small microwave-safe bowl, whisk together the peanut butter, water, and vanilla (the mixture doesn't have to be completely smooth). Microwave on high for 30 to 45 seconds, or until the mixture bubbles and starts to thicken. Remove from the microwave and stir until smooth. Add the chocolate chips and stir just to coat; do not stir until melted. Pour the sauce over the banana slices and serve immediately.

Per serving: Protein: 3g • Calories: 141 • Dietary Fiber: 1g

Pear-Chai Pudding

The flavors of chai tea—cinnamon, cardamom, cloves, nutmeg, and other spices—give this pudding an exotic taste.

Makes 4 servings

2 cups nonfat milk

1 package (4-serving size) sugar-free vanilla instant custard mix

1 double-spice chai tea bag

1 large pear

4 teaspoons sliced almonds, toasted

Put the milk into a medium saucepan and whisk in the pudding mix. Add the tea bag. Cook over medium heat, stirring constantly, taking care not to break the tea bag. Remove the tea bag after 2 minutes. Continue cooking and stirring until the mixture comes to a full boil. Divide the pudding among four serving bowls. Cover each bowl with plastic wrap; the wrap should be directly touching the pudding so a skin doesn't form. Chill for at least 2 hours. Remove the plastic wrap. Top each bowl with some diced pear and toasted almonds before serving.

Per serving: Protein: 5g • Calories: 110 • Dietary Fiber: 2g

Pumpkin-Oat Cookies

Makes 18 cookies; 2 per serving

5 tablespoons canned pumpkin puree (not pumpkin pie filling)

2 tablespoons unsalted butter, softened, or coconut oil

½ cup whole wheat pancake mix

2 (1-ounce) envelopes no-sugar-added, cinnamon-flavored instant oats (slightly rounded ½ cup)

¼ cup orange marmalade all-fruit spread

2 tablespoons sliced almonds or mini chocolate chips (optional)

Preheat the oven to 350°F. Line a baking sheet with parchment paper or spray it with nonstick cooking spray.

In a mixing bowl, cream the pumpkin and butter until well blended. Add the pancake mix and oats, stirring just until the mixture begins to hold together. Do not overmix. Stir in the marmalade and nuts just until blended. Drop the batter by level tablespoons close together on the prepared baking sheet; flatten each with a fork. The cookies won't spread.

Bake for 15 to 20 minutes, until the cookies are golden brown. Remove from the oven and let cool on the baking sheet for 5 minutes before removing them to wire rack to cool completely.

Per serving: Protein: 2g • Calories: 92 • Dietary Fiber: 1g

Raspberry Meringue Dessert

Makes 6 servings

1 package (4-serving size) sugar-free vanilla instant pudding mix

2 cups nonfat milk

⅔ cup nonfat plain Greek yogurt

1 cup fresh raspberries, coarsely chopped

10 sugar-free mini vanilla meringue cookies

Prepare the pudding as directed on the package, using nonfat milk. Fold in the yogurt and raspberries. Just before serving, coarsely crumble the meringues into the pudding mixture. (The meringues will melt if added ahead of time.) Divide the mixture among six serving dishes. Serve immediately.

Per serving: Protein: 5g • Calories: 72 • Dietary Fiber: 2g

Strawberry Cheesecake Mousse

Makes 4 servings

1 cup fat-free cottage cheese

1 package (4-serving size) sugar-free instant cheesecake pudding
  mix

¾ cup nonfat plain Greek yogurt

1 cup sliced strawberries

Put the cottage cheese in a small food processor or blender. Blend until smooth, about 1 minute. Add the pudding mix and process until combined. Add the yogurt and pulse just until well blended. Pour the mixture into a medium bowl. Fold in the strawberries. Divide the mixture among four bowls and serve immediately, or chill until serving time.

Per serving: Protein: 6g • Calories: 102 • Dietary Fiber: 1g

Pineapple-Coconut Cupcakes

Makes 24 servings

1 (20-ounce) can pineapple chunks in juice, drained, juice reserved

1 (16-ounce) box sugar-free yellow cake mix

4 large egg whites

⅓ cup nonfat plain Greek yogurt

1 tablespoon imitation coconut or rum extract

Preheat the oven to 325°F. Line 24 muffin cups with foil liners, or spray paper liners with nonstick cooking spray. Place a scant table-spoon of pineapple chunks (about six chunks each) into lined muffin cups. Put the cake mix into the bowl of a standing mixer. Add 1 cup of the reserved pineapple juice (adding water to make 1 cup, if needed) along with the egg whites, yogurt, and coconut extract. Beat on medium speed for 2 minutes; pour ¼ cup of the batter into each muffin cup. Bake as package directs, 19 to 23 minutes. The cupcakes are done when a toothpick inserted into the center comes out clean. Cool in the pan for 10 to 15 minutes before removing to a wire rack to cool completely.

Per serving: Protein: 2g • Calories: 78 • Dietary Fiber: 1g

Apple Chips

The final yield on these oven-roasted fruit chips will depend upon how thickly you slice your apples and in what shapes. Smaller cuts (such as from a quartered apple) will dry into smaller pieces, while larger slices (from the entire diameter of the fruit) will make larger chips. You also can make this treat with pears.

Makes 4 servings

2 large apples, washed and cored, halved or left whole

Ground cinnamon, to taste

Preheat the oven to 225°F. Line two baking sheets with nonstick baking mats or parchment paper.

Using a mandoline or a knife, cut the whole or halved apples into very thin slices. Arrange the slices in a single layer on the lined baking sheets and bake undisturbed for 1 hour. Remove the sheets from the oven and carefully turn the slices with a thin spatula. Sprinkle the tops lightly with cinnamon, if desired, and bake for 1 more hour. Turn off the heat and let the chips finish drying in the oven, 20 to 30 minutes, depending upon their thickness.

Let cool completely on the baking sheets. Transfer to an airtight container and store at room temperature for up to 1 week.

Per serving: Protein: 0g • Calories: 39 • Dietary Fiber: 1g

Melon Ribbons

Served cold, these ribbons make a simple dessert. Or quickly warmed through in a large nonstick skillet over low heat, they make a sweet "pasta" pairing for seafood topped with Mango Salsa (page 289). For a particularly beautiful presentation, serve a mix of sweet melon varieties with ribbons of different colors.

Makes 4 servings

1 melon, peeled, halved, and seeds removed, or a combination of melons

1 tablespoon fresh lime juice (optional)

½ cup Orange-Mint Yogurt Sauce (page 284) (optional)

Cut each melon half into quarters and, using a vegetable peeler or mandoline, cut ribbons as thin as possible from the sides. Place the ribbons in a bowl and toss with the lime juice, if desired. Cover and chill until ready to serve. Arrange the ribbons decoratively on plates and serve with the yogurt sauce, if you like. (The melon ribbons will keep, covered and refrigerated, for up to 2 days.)

Per serving: Protein: 3g • Calories: 66 • Dietary Fiber: 1g

Roasted Peaches

Roasted or grilled stone fruit make a terrific accompaniment to meat. Or you can stuff the centers of these with frozen blueberries or raspberries for a filling dessert. All stone fruits are delicious when roasted—try this same method with pitted apricots, cherries, plums, and nectarines, adjusting the cooking time accordingly.

Makes 4 servings

Vegetable oil spray

4 peaches, skin on, halved and pitted

¼ teaspoon ground cinnamon

¼ cup frozen or fresh blueberries or raspberries (optional)

½ cup Orange-Mint Yogurt Sauce (page 284) (optional)

Preheat the oven to 400°F. Line a baking sheet with aluminum foil and lightly spray with vegetable oil spray.

Place the peaches, cut sides up, on the baking sheet and lightly sprinkle the top of each half with a pinch of the cinnamon. Roast cut sides down until the fruits start to become tender, 12 to 15 minutes. Turn and continue roasting until completely tender, 5 to 8 minutes, filling the centers of each half with the berries, if desired, during this time. Serve hot or warm, topping each half with 1 tablespoon of yogurt sauce, if desired.

Per serving: Protein: 3g • Calories: 79 • Dietary Fiber: 3g

SAUCES AND CONDIMENTS

When you're enjoying your all-you-can-eat snacks, why not add a little extra flavor to the mix? The Age-Defying Diet works not only because of my research behind it, but because the SuperCharged Smoothies, SuperCharged Soups, and whole-food meals are healthy and delicious, which keeps you right on track for a fit figure. Why not try adding Pesto to chicken or shrimp, or topping some Courgette Noodles with Tomato Sauce to boost their flavors? This can help curb your appetite, because your food is more satisfying. Weight loss problems arise when commercial condiments, such as pesto with a lot of cheese and olive oil or tomato sauce with high-fructose corn syrup, are used with abandon.

Here are some recipes for sauces and condiments that you can mix and match with main courses, vegetables, grains, and snacks. Spoon some Lemon-Artichoke Sauce over Tabbouleh or serve it with whole steamed artichokes. Pair Pico de Gallo with grilled chicken breasts. Serve some Tzatziki with blanched vegetables. Whenever you add a sauce or a condiment, limit yourself to one serving per meal. The possibilities are endless. You will find more sauce and condiment recipes on my website DrApovian.com. And download the Age-Defying Coach app. It's free with this book (see page 294).

Dijon Mustard Lemon Dressing

Make this your go-to dressing for tossing salad greens or drizzling over steamed vegetables—artichokes, asparagus, broccoli, carrots, you name it. You can also double this recipe. Put twice the amount of ingredients in a jar, cover, and give it a good shake before using.

Makes ⅓ cup; 1 tablespoon per serving

2½ teaspoons Dijon mustard

2 teaspoons fresh lemon juice

1 teaspoon minced shallots or onions

⅛ teaspoon salt

⅛ teaspoon ground black pepper

2 teaspoons extra-virgin olive oil

¼ cup canned vegetable stock

Place the mustard, lemon juice, shallots, salt, and pepper in a small bowl and whisk to combine. Add the oil and whisk to combine. Whisking, slowly drizzle in the stock 2 teaspoons at a time, until it has all been added and the mixture is frothy and well combined. Serve at room temperature or cold on salads. (The dressing will keep, tightly covered and refrigerated, for up to 2 days. Whisk before using.)

Per serving: Protein: 0g • Calories: 24 • Dietary Fiber: 0g

Mayonnaise

While the flavor of this isn't *exactly* like that of real mayonnaise, it comes pretty close. It is a good dip on its own, and has the added bonus of calcium and protein without the fat calories.

This also makes a great base for other dips and salads, including the Waldorf Salad and Waldorf Chicken Salad (page 244). You can jazz this up by adding chopped spring onions, dill, parsley, garlic, and a pinch of cayenne.

Makes about 2 cups; 2 tablespoons per serving

1⅓ cups nonfat Greek yogurt

2 tablespoons nonfat mayonnaise

2 teaspoons fresh lemon juice

1 teaspoon Dijon mustard

1 teaspoon extra-virgin olive oil

¼ teaspoon paprika

¼ teaspoon salt

Whisk together all of the ingredients in a bowl until smooth. Cover and refrigerate for up to 4 days.

Per serving: Protein: 2g • Calories: 21 • Dietary Fiber: 0g

Lemon-Artichoke Sauce

The bright flavors of this sauce go with many proteins—chicken, pork or veal, tofu, shrimp, or fish. It's also a lively topping for pasta, vegetables, and whole grains. By using frozen artichoke hearts, this recipe comes together in minutes. Defrost the hearts in the package at room temperature while you gather the other ingredients.

Makes about 3 cups; ½ cup per serving

1 teaspoon extra-virgin olive oil

1 tablespoon chopped shallots or onions

½ teaspoon crushed garlic

½ teaspoon chopped fresh thyme or a pinch of dried thyme

¼ teaspoon ground black pepper

¼ teaspoon salt

6 teaspoons dry white wine

2 tablespoons fresh lemon juice

½ teaspoon finely grated lemon zest

½ cup canned low-sodium chicken stock or vegetable stock

1 (9-ounce) package frozen artichoke hearts, thawed

1½ teaspoons chopped fresh parsley

Heat the oil in a large nonstick skillet over medium-high heat. Add the shallots and cook, stirring, until soft, about 1 minute. Add the garlic, thyme, pepper, and salt, and cook, stirring, until fragrant, 20 to 30 seconds. Add the white wine and cook until nearly evaporated, 30 to 45 seconds. Stir in the lemon juice and zest. Immediately add the stock, bring to the boil, and boil for 30 seconds. Add the artichoke hearts and return to the boil. Lower the heat and simmer undisturbed until the hearts are tender and cooked through, 3 to 5 minutes. Stir in the parsley and serve immediately.

Per serving: Protein: 1g • Calories: 31 • Dietary Fiber: 2g

Orange-Mint Yogurt Sauce

Use this light topping on the Berry-Spinach Frittata (page 235) or as a dip for fresh fruit or steamed broccoli, cauliflower, or asparagus (page 245). Make this only with fresh orange juice you squeeze yourself; do not use packaged juice, which often has added sugar and calories.

Makes ¾ cup; 2 tablespoons per serving

½ cup nonfat Greek yogurt

4 teaspoons fresh orange juice

1 tablespoon chopped fresh mint

½ teaspoon finely grated orange zest

3 tablespoons peeled and seeded fresh orange segments, cut into ½-inch pieces

Stir together the yogurt, juice, mint, and zest in a small bowl. Fold in the orange pieces. Serve immediately, or cover and refrigerate until ready to serve. (The sauce will keep, covered and refrigerated, for up to 1 day. Stir before serving.)

Per serving: Protein: 2g • Calories: 20 • Dietary Fiber: 0g

Raspberry-Balsamic Sauce

Drizzle a couple of tablespoons of this sauce over grilled chicken breasts or boneless pork chops.

Makes about 1 cup; 2 tablespoons per serving

½ teaspoon extra-virgin olive oil

2 tablespoons chopped shallots or onions

¼ cup white balsamic vinegar

2 cups fresh or frozen raspberries, thawed

Stevia or other sugar substitute, to taste

Heat the oil in a medium skillet over medium heat. Add the shallots and cook, stirring, until soft, 1 to 1½ minutes. Add the vinegar and cook undisturbed until reduced by half, 1 to 1½ minutes. Add the raspberries and cook, stirring, until falling apart, about 2 minutes. Remove from the heat and transfer to a blender. Puree the mixture and adjust the seasoning to taste with sugar substitute. Strain through a fine-mesh strainer into a clean bowl; discard the solids in the strainer. (The sauce will keep, tightly covered and refrigerated, for up to 4 days.)

Per serving: Protein: 0g • Calories: 27 • Dietary Fiber: 2g

Pesto

This version of the classic Italian sauce, made with mixed herbs, is missing the fat, but not the flavor. Spoon some onto pasta, rice, fish, chicken, or pork. If you prefer, you can make it with just one herb. Remove the leaves from the herb, discard the stems, and then wash and dry them thoroughly before using.

Makes 1 cup; 2 tablespoons per serving

2 packed cups fresh basil leaves

2 packed cups fresh parsley leaves

1 packed cup fresh mint leaves

2½ teaspoons fresh lemon juice

2 teaspoons toasted walnuts, pine nuts, or pecans

¼ cup crushed garlic

¼ teaspoon salt

½ teaspoon ground black pepper

1 tablespoon extra-virgin olive oil

Place the basil, parsley, mint, lemon juice, nuts, garlic, salt, and pepper in a food processor and process on high speed until the ingredients are finely chopped and well combined, scraping down the sides of the bowl as needed. Add the olive oil and process to a fine paste, again scraping down the sides as needed to incorporate all the ingredients.

Serve at room temperature as a sauce or seasoning blend. (The pesto will keep in an airtight container, refrigerated, for up to 3 days. Stir well before using.)

Per serving: Protein: 1g • Calories: 35 • Dietary Fiber: 1g

Tomato Sauce

This savory sauce can be served as a topping to just about everything—from fish and chicken to pasta and rice. It's delicious, too, on vegetables, such as the Courgette Torte (page 237).

Makes 3 cups; ½ cup per serving

1 teaspoon extra-virgin olive oil

½ cup chopped onions

¼ cup chopped carrots

¼ cup chopped celery

1¼ teaspoons chopped garlic

¼ teaspoon salt

¼ teaspoon ground black pepper

1 bay leaf

2 (14½-ounce) cans chopped tomatoes and their juice

1 tablespoon chopped fresh basil or 1 teaspoon dried basil

2 teaspoons chopped fresh oregano or ½ teaspoon dried oregano

2 teaspoons chopped fresh parsley or 1 teaspoon dried parsley

Heat the oil in a medium pot over medium-high heat. Add the onions, carrots, and celery and cook, stirring, until soft, about 4 minutes. Add the garlic, salt, pepper, and bay leaf, and cook, stirring, until fragrant, 30 to 45 seconds. Add the tomatoes and their juices, stir, and bring to the boil. Reduce the heat and simmer, uncovered, until the mixture is slightly reduced, 12 to 14 minutes. Add the herbs and cook until fragrant, about 1½ minutes.

Remove the sauce from the heat and puree with a handheld blender, or in two batches in a food processor.

Serve hot. (The sauce can be made ahead and kept, refrigerated, in an airtight container, for up to 5 days, or frozen for up to 1 month. Reheat gently over low heat and serve hot.)

Per serving: Protein: 1g • Calories: 40 • Dietary Fiber: 2g

Tzatziki

This tangy Greek yogurt sauce makes a flavorful partner for roasted, grilled, or sautéed fish and chicken. It also is a delicious dip for raw or cooked vegetables.

Makes 1½ cups; 2 tablespoons per serving

1 cup nonfat plain Greek yogurt

½ cup peeled, deseeded, and finely chopped cucumber

2 teaspoons extra-virgin olive oil

1½ teaspoons fresh lemon juice

¾ teaspoon chopped fresh dill or ¼ teaspoon dried dill

½ teaspoon crushed garlic, or more to taste

¼ teaspoon salt

Pinch of paprika

Whisk together all of the ingredients in a medium bowl. Cover and refrigerate for at least 1 hour to allow the flavors to marry. (The sauce can be kept, covered, in the refrigerator for up to 3 days.)

Per serving: Protein: 2g • Calories: 20 • Dietary Fiber: 0g

Mango Salsa

This colorful fruit salsa can be made to suit your tastes and the seasonality of your favorite fruits. Mix and match to create new flavors—for instance, you could try peaches and nectarines, mango and papaya, or mango and pineapple. This recipe also can be made with frozen fruit. Thaw the fruit at room temperature and blot dry with towels before using to enjoy the flavors of summer all year long.

Makes about 2½ cups; ½ cup per serving

2 cups peeled, stoned, and chopped fresh or frozen mangoes (about 2 large) or other fruit

3 tablespoons stoned and chopped red or yellow pepper

3 tablespoons chopped red onions

2 tablespoons fresh lime juice

4 teaspoons sliced spring onions

4 teaspoons deseeded and chopped jalapeños

2 teaspoons chopped fresh coriander

Put all the ingredients in a large bowl and gently stir to combine. Serve at room temperature, or cover and refrigerate until ready to serve. (The salsa will keep for up to 2 days, covered, in the refrigerator.)

Per serving: Protein: 1g • Calories: 50 • Dietary Fiber: 2g

Pico de Gallo

Serve this Mexican salsa with grilled or roasted chicken breasts, vegetables, Boiled Shrimp (page 233), or grilled fish.

Makes a generous 2 cups; ½ cup per serving

1½ cups deseeded and chopped tomatoes

½ cup chopped onions

3 tablespoons chopped fresh coriander

2 tablespoons fresh lime juice

1 tablespoon plus 1 teaspoon deseeded and chopped fresh jalapeños

1 teaspoon crushed garlic

¼ teaspoon salt

Combine all the ingredients in a medium bowl and mix well. Serve at room temperature, or cover and refrigerate until ready to serve. (The sauce will keep, covered and refrigerated, for up to 2 days.)

Per serving: Protein: 1g • Calories: 25 • Dietary Fiber: 1g

Gremolata

A sprinkle of this flavorful blend of lemon zest, garlic, and parsley is most frequently used as a condiment for the classic Italian dish osso buco. Add some to Courgette Noodles (page 255), chicken or fish cooked in foil packets (pages 215, 230), or on steamed or roasted vegetables (pages 245, 246).

Makes heaping ¼ cup; 1 tablespoon per serving

¼ cup chopped fresh parsley

2 teaspoons finely grated lemon zest

2 teaspoons crushed garlic

⅛ teaspoon salt, or to taste

Pinch of ground black pepper, or to taste

Blend the ingredients in a small bowl. Use immediately. (The gremolata will keep, tightly covered and refrigerated, for up to 2 days.)

Per serving: Protein: 0g • Calories: 8 • Dietary Fiber: 1g

Roasted Garlic

Roasting garlic reduces its pungency and gives it a milder, sweet flavor. Roasting also softens the cloves, making it easy to mash them into a paste to flavor sauces and dips. Add some to vegetables or soups for another layer of flavor. The yield will depend on how large the garlic heads are.

Makes about ¼ cup; 1 tablespoon per serving

2 heads garlic, top one-quarter sliced from each to expose the cloves

1½ teaspoons extra-virgin olive oil

4 teaspoons water

Pinch of salt

Pinch of ground black pepper

Preheat the oven to 325°F. Place a 10 x 10-inch piece of aluminum foil on a baking sheet.

Place the garlic, cut sides up, in the center of the foil. Drizzle the cut cloves of each with ¾ teaspoon of the oil, 2 teaspoons of the water, and the salt and pepper. Wrap the foil around the garlic, pressing to seal, and roast until the garlic is soft to the touch and fragrant, 45 minutes to 1 hour.

Remove from the oven, unwrap, and let rest until cool enough to handle. Squeeze the cloves from the skins into a small bowl and leave whole or mash into a paste. (The cloves will keep, tightly covered, in the refrigerator for up to 5 days.)

Per serving: Protein: 1g • Calories: 28 • Dietary Fiber: 0g

Whole Wheat Bread Crumbs

Fresh homemade bread crumbs are a step above the usual commercial varieties in terms of both flavor and texture. Bread crumbs are used in the Courgette Torte (page 237) and the Turkey Meat Loaf (page 225), and sprinkling 1 tablespoon on top of steamed vegetables adds a nice crunch. Remember that one slice of whole wheat or whole-grain bread constitutes one daily serving. Each slice of bread will make about ⅔ cup of crumbs, so measure these out and use accordingly.

Makes 1⅓ cups; 2 tablespoons per serving

1 slice commercially made whole wheat or whole-grain bread, cut
   into ¾-inch cubes

Preheat the oven to 250°F. Line a large baking sheet with aluminum foil or parchment paper.

Place the bread cubes in a food processor and process on high speed into fine crumbs, about 1 minute. Place the crumbs on the baking sheet, spreading evenly to the edges, and bake for 10 minutes. Stir the crumbs and continue baking until fragrant, completely dry, and very lightly toasted, 15 to 20 minutes. Remove from the oven and let cool completely before using. (Bread crumbs can be stored in an airtight container at room temperature for up to 10 days.)

Per serving: Protein: 1g • Calories: 14g • Dietary Fiber: 0g

Your Age-Defying Coach

I created the Age-Defying Coach first for my patients and now for you. Access it digitally via your desktop, smartphone, laptop, or tablet to keep the momentum going whenever, wherever! I offer it to you free of charge, because your success is as important to me as the success of my patients. I have devoted my entire medical career to helping people just like you (and me) lose weight, and I know a little extra help never hurts. Besides, it's always nice to have a buddy when you're making a life change; think of the Age-Defying Coach as your virtual trainer, friend, and source of inspiration, without the cost of a personal trainer! The Age-Defying Coach has tools to help you every step of the way—tracking and planning tools to help you outsmart your metabolism, lose weight, and look and feel younger. When you use it as little as 30 seconds each day, you will receive my helpful, constructive feedback for each step in the diet, and beyond. My patients love it, and I think you will, too. Just come to my website DrApovian.com, go to Age-Defying Coach, and sign in using this password:

AgeDefying101

Here's a brief summary of just some of the tools I have for you:

- **Color My Day Applet** asks that you assess how you're feeling about reaching your goals with nothing more than a gut reaction, using colors to track your daily progress. Use green when you feel that you're right on track (you're eating, exercising, and sleeping healthily); red when you go off the rails (ate pizza and a hot fudge sundae)—hey, it happens to the best of us sometimes (even me), so don't be too hard on yourself; and yellow when it's a mixed bag (for example, plenty of vegetables but not enough protein that day).

By doing this every day, you send a subtle message to yourself that you are committed to developing healthy behaviors and support the process of change. (People who log in a color at least five out of each seven days get the best results.) Trust me, patterns will emerge on your calendar that you didn't realize were happening. As a result, you'll be able to make significant changes in what you eat and how you exercise that will get your metabolism moving. The Coach lets you send yourself a text reminder each day to evaluate your day in this way; when you reply to the text, your calendar is automatically updated.

• **Activity Applet** allows you to set your goals, and then track your weight, the number of steps walked, minutes of physical activity, and other metrics. You can even send yourself an automated text at a specific delivery time you choose to remind you that, say, a strength-training class at the gym starts in 45 minutes. If you use a Fitbit or UP activity tracker, you can pair these devices with your Age-Defying Coach and your activities will automatically be updated.

• **Journaling Applet** is an online diary tool that lets you record anything you feel is relevant about your journey to optimum health. Journaling is sometimes referred to as "bibliotherapy," and there is a good deal of scientific research that shows how effective it is in promoting positive behavior change. And without all the fancy terminology, getting out your feelings on paper is always a good way to stay sane and remind yourself why you're committed to changing your body for good.

• **Planning Applet** allows you to create a custom eating plan and shopping lists. You can include meals from this book plus scores of others. Like the Activity Applet, the Planning Applet allows you to send yourself text reminders to help you stick to your plan.

Stay in Touch

My readers are as important to me as my patients. Don't hesitate to reach out to me on Facebook, Twitter, Pinterest, Google Plus, Instagram, or my website DrApovian.com with any questions or just to brag about how much weight you have lost and how much younger you look and feel. You're the reason I wrote this book, so you can have a healthier and happier life. When I was in college, I packed on the pounds. Desperate to lose weight like so many people, I found the secret to permanent weight loss. You can do the same. Take back your life, vitality, and waistline.

APPENDIX A

Converting to Metrics

Volume Measurement Conversions

U.S.	Metric
¼ teaspoon	1.25 ml
½ teaspoon	2.5 ml
¾ teaspoon	3.75 ml
1 teaspoon	5 ml
1 tablespoon	15 ml
¼ cup	62.5 ml
½ cup	125 ml
¾ cup	187.5 ml
1 cup	250 ml

Weight Conversion Measurements

U.S.	Metric
1 ounce	28.4 g
8 ounces	227.5 g
16 ounces (1 pound)	455 g

Cooking Temperature Conversions

Celsius/Centigrade	0°C and 100°C are arbitrarily placed at the melting and boiling points of water and standard to the metric system.
Fahrenheit	Fahrenheit established 0°F as the stabilized temperature when equal amounts of ice, water, and salt are mixed.

To convert temperatures in Fahrenheit to Celsius, use this formula:

$$C = (F-32) \times 0.5555$$

So, for example, if you are baking at 350°F and want to know that temperature in Celsius, use this calculation:

$$C = (350-32) \times 0.5555 = 176.66°C$$

APPENDIX B

Find Your BMI

Find your height in the left-hand column, then find your weight in the row above. Your BMI is at the intersection of your height and weight.

		Weight (lb)										
		120	**130**	**140**	**150**	**160**	**170**	**180**	**190**	**200**	**210**	**220**
	4'5"	30	33	35	38	40	43	45	48	50	53	55
	4'6"	29	31	34	36	39	41	43	46	48	51	53
	4'7"	28	30	33	35	27	40	42	44	47	49	51
	4'8"	27	29	31	34	36	38	40	43	45	47	49
	4'9"	26	28	30	33	35	37	39	41	43	46	48
	4'10"	25	27	29	31	34	36	38	40	42	44	46
	4'11"	24	26	28	30	32	34	36	38	40	43	45
	5'0"	23	25	27	29	31	33	35	37	39	41	43
	5'1"	23	25	27	28	30	32	34	36	38	40	42
	5'2"	22	24	26	27	29	31	33	35	37	38	40
	5'3"	21	23	25	27	28	30	32	34	36	37	39
Height (ft/in)	**5'4"**	21	22	24	26	28	29	31	33	34	36	38
	5'5"	20	22	23	25	27	28	30	32	33	35	37
	5'6"	19	21	23	24	26	27	29	31	32	34	36
	5'7"	19	20	22	24	25	27	28	30	31	33	35
	5'8"	18	20	21	23	24	26	27	29	30	32	34
	5'9"	18	19	21	22	24	25	27	28	30	31	33
	5'10"	17	19	20	22	23	24	26	27	29	30	32
	5'11"	17	18	20	21	22	24	25	27	28	29	31
	6'0"	16	18	19	20	22	23	24	26	27	29	30
	6'1"	16	17	19	20	21	22	24	25	26	28	29
	6'2"	15	17	18	19	21	22	23	24	26	27	28
	6'3"	15	16	18	19	20	21	23	24	25	26	28
	6'4"	15	16	17	18	20	21	22	23	24	26	27
	6'5"	14	15	17	18	19	20	21	23	24	25	26
	6'6"	14	15	16	17	19	20	21	22	23	24	25
	6'7"	14	15	16	17	18	19	20	21	23	24	25
	6'8"	13	14	15	17	18	19	20	21	22	23	24

Weight (lb)												
230	240	250	260	270	280	290	300	310	320	330	340	350
58	60	63	65	68	70	73	75	78	80	83	85	88
56	58	60	63	65	68	70	72	75	77	80	82	84
54	56	58	61	63	65	68	70	72	75	77	79	81
52	54	56	58	61	63	65	68	70	72	74	76	79
50	52	54	56	59	61	63	65	67	69	72	74	76
48	50	52	54	57	59	61	63	65	67	69	71	73
47	49	51	53	55	57	59	61	63	65	67	69	71
45	47	49	51	53	55	57	59	61	63	65	66	68
44	45	47	49	51	53	55	57	59	61	62	64	66
42	44	46	48	49	51	53	55	57	59	60	62	64
41	43	44	46	48	50	51	53	55	57	59	60	62
40	41	43	45	46	48	50	52	53	55	57	58	60
38	40	42	43	45	47	48	50	52	53	55	57	58
37	39	40	42	44	45	47	49	50	52	53	55	57
36	38	39	41	42	44	46	47	49	50	52	53	55
35	37	38	40	41	43	44	46	47	49	50	52	53
34	36	37	38	40	41	43	44	46	47	49	50	52
33	35	36	37	39	40	42	43	45	46	47	49	50
32	34	35	36	38	39	41	42	43	45	46	47	49
31	33	34	35	37	38	39	41	42	43	45	46	48
30	32	33	34	36	37	38	40	41	42	44	45	46
30	31	32	33	35	36	37	39	40	41	42	44	45
29	30	31	33	34	35	36	38	39	40	41	43	44
28	29	30	32	33	34	35	37	38	39	40	41	43
27	29	30	31	32	33	34	36	37	38	39	40	42
27	28	29	30	31	32	34	35	36	37	38	39	40
26	27	28	29	30	32	33	34	35	36	37	38	39
25	26	28	29	30	31	32	33	34	35	36	37	38

References

Anderson, A. L., Harris, T. B., Tylavsky, F. A., et al. (2011). Dietary patterns and survival of older adults. *Journal of the American Dietetic Association, 111*(1), 84–91.

Apovian, C. M., & Aronne, L. J. (2013, August 14). Zonisamide for weight reduction in obese adults. *Journal of the American Medical Association, 310*(6), 637–638.

Apovian, C. M., & Aronne, L. J. (2013, December 18). Weight loss treatment in obese adults—reply. *Journal of the American Medical Association, 310*(23), 2568.

Apovian, C. M., Frey, C. M., Heydt, D., et al. (2002). Body mass index and physical function in older women. *Obesity Research, 10*(8), 740–747.

Apovian, C. M., & Gokce, N. (2012). Obesity and cardiovascular disease. *Circulation, 125*(9), 1178–1182. PMCID: PMC3693443.

Apovian, C. M., & Korner, J. (2012). Proven weight loss methods. *Journal of Clinical Endocrinology and Metabolism, 97*(7), A33–4.

Apovian, C. M., & Mechanick, J. I. (2010). Disrupting the food-fat connection. *Current Opinion in Endocrinology, Diabetes and Obesity, 17,* 440.

Apovian, C. M., & Mechanick, J. I. (2013, October). Obesity IS a disease! *Current Opinion in Endocrinology, Diabetes and Obesity, 20*(5), 367–368.

Artero, E. G., Lee, D. C., Lavie, C. J., et al. (2012). Effects of muscular strength on cardiovascular risk factors and prognosis. *Journal of Cardiopulmonary Rehabilitation and Prevention, 32*(6), 351–58. http://dx.doi.org/10.1097/HCR. 0b013e3182642688.

Astrup, A., Dyerberg, J., Elwood, P., et al. (2011). The role of reducing intakes of saturated fat in the prevention of cardiovascular disease: Where does the evidence stand in 2010? *American Journal of Clinical Nutrition, 93*(4), 684–688.

Barone Gibbs, B., Kinzel, L. S., Pettee Gabriel, K., et al. (2012). Short-term and long-term eating habit modification predicts weight change in overweight, postmenopausal women: Results from the WOMAN study. *Journal of the Academy of Nutrition and Dietetics, 112*(9), 1347–1355. http://dx.doi.org/10.1016/j.jand. 2012.06.012.

Basaria, S., Coviello, A. D., Travison, T. G., et al. (2010). Adverse events associated with testosterone administration. *New England Journal of Medicine, 363,* 109–122. http://dx.doi.org/10.1056/NEJMoa1000485.

Bigornia, S. J., Farb, M. G., Tiwari, S., Karki, S., Hamburg, N. M., Vita, J. A., Hess, D. T., Lavalley, M. P., Apovian, C. M., & Gokce, N. (2013, December 17). Insulin status and vascular responses to weight loss in obesity. *Journal of the American College of Cardiology, 62*(24), 2297–2305. PMCID: PMC3873767.

Bistrian, B. R., Winterer, J. C., Blackburn, G. L., et al. (1977). Failure of yellow fever immunization to produce a catabolic response in individuals fully adapted to a protein-sparing modified fast. *American Journal of Clinical Nutrition, 30,* 1518–1522.

Bjermo, H., Iggam, D., Kullberg, J., et al. (2012). Effects of n-6 PUFAs compared with SFAs on liver fat, lipoproteins, and inflammation in abdominal obesity: A randomized controlled trial. *American Journal of Clinical Nutrition, 95*(5), 1003–1012. http://dx.doi.org/10.3945/ajcn.111.030114.

Blackburn, G. L., Hutter, M. M., Harvey, A. M., Apovian, C. M., Boulton, H. R., Cummings, S., Fallon, J. A., Greenberg, I., Jiser, M. E., Jones, D. B., Jones, S. B., Kaplan, L. M., Kelly, J. J., Kruger, R. S. Jr., Lautz, D. B., Lenders, C. M., Lonigro, R., Luce, H., McNamara, A., Mulligan, A. T., Paasche-Orlow, M. K., Perna, F. M., Pratt, J. S., Riley, S. M. Jr., Robinson, M. K., Romanelli, J. R., Saltzman, E., Schumann, R., Shikora, S. A., Snow, R. L., Sogg, S., Sullivan, M. A., Tarnoff, M., Thompson, C. C., Wee, C. C., Ridley, N., Auerbach, J., Hu, F. B., Kirle, L., Buckley, R. B., & Annas, C. L. (2009). Expert panel on weight loss surgery: Executive report update. *Obesity (Silver Spring), 17*(5), 842–862.

Blackburn, G. L., Phillips, J. C. C., & Morreale, S. (2001). Physicians' guide to popular low-carbohydrate weight-loss diets. *Cleveland Clinic Journal of Medicine, 68,* 751.

Blom, W. A. M., Lluch, A., Stafleu, A., et al. (2006). Effect of a high-protein breakfast on the postprandial ghrelin response. *American Journal of Clinical Nutrition, 83,* 211–220.

Boyle, T., Bull, F., Fritschi, L., et al. (2012). Resistance training and the risk of colon and rectal cancers. *Cancer Causes and Control, 23,* 1091–1097. http://dx.doi.org/10.1007/s10552-012-9978-x.

Breslau, N. A., Brinkley, L., Hill, K. D., et al. (1988). Relationship of animal protein-rich diet to kidney stone formation and calcium metabolism. *Journal of Clinical Endocrinology and Metabolism, 66*(1), 140–146. http://dx.doi.org/10.1210/jcem-66-1-140.

Brooks, N., Layne, J., Gordon, P., et al. (2006). Strength training improves muscle quality and insulin sensitivity in older Hispanics with type 2 diabetes. *Diabetes Care, 4*(1), 19–27.

Broussard, J. L., Ehrmann, D. A., Van Cauter, E., et al. (2012). Impaired insulin signaling in human adipocytes after experimental sleep restriction: A randomized, crossover study. *Annals of Internal Medicine, 157*(8), 549–557. http://dx.doi.org/10.7326/0003-4819-157-8-201210160-00005.

Brown, A. B., McCartney, N., & Sale, D. G. (1990). Positive adaptations to weight-lifting training in elderly adults. *Journal of Applied Physiology, 69,* 1725–1733.

Brown, J. M., Yetter, J. F., Spicer, M. J., et al. (1978). Cardiac complications of protein-sparing modified fast. *Journal of the American Medical Association, 240,* 120–122.

Campbell, W. W., Trappe, T. A., Wolfe, R. R., et al. (2001). The recommended dietary allowance for protein may not be adequate for older people to maintain healthy skeletal muscle. *Journals of Gerontology Series A: Biological Sciences and Medical Sciences, 56,* M373–380.

Casperson, S. L., Sheffield-Moore, M., Hewlings, S. J., et al. (2012). Leucine supplementation chronically improves muscle protein synthesis in older adults consuming the RDA for protein. *Clinical Nutrition, 31*(4), 512–519. http://dx.doi.org/10.1016/j.clnu.2012.01.005.

Cassilhas, R. C., Fernandes, J., Oliveira, M. G. M., et al. (2010, November 13–17). The impact of 8 weeks of aerobic or resistance exercise on spatial memory and hippocampal BDNF of rodents. Paper presented at the 40th Society for Neuroscience Annual Meeting, San Diego, CA.

Castaneda, C., Charnley, J. M., Evans, W. J., et al. (1995). Elderly women accommodate to a low-protein diet with losses of body cell mass, muscle function, and immune response. *American Journal of Clinical Nutrition, 62,* 30–39.

Centers for Disease Control and Prevention. (2013). Adult participation in aerobic and muscle-strengthening physical activities—United States, 2011. *Morbidity and Mortality Weekly Report, 62*(17), 326–330.

Cho, E., Speigelman, D., Hunter, D. J., et al. (2003). Premenopausal fat intake and risk of breast cancer. *Journal of the National Cancer Institute, 95,* 1079–1085.

Cire, B. (2010, June 30). Adverse cardiovascular events reported in testosterone trial in older men: Treatment phase of clinical trial halted. National Institute on Aging. *Cochrane Database for Systematic Reviews, 6*(7), CD000333. http://dx.doi.org/10.1002/14651858.CD000333.pub2.

Clifton, P. (2006). The science behind weight loss diets: A brief review. *Australian Family Physician, 35*(8), 580–582.

Cohen, P. G. (2008). Obesity in men: The hypogonadal-estrogen receptor relationship and its effect on glucose homeostasis. *Medical Hypotheses, 70*(2), 358–360.

A critique of low-carbohydrate ketogenic weight reduction regimens: A review of *Dr. Atkins' Diet Revolution.* (1974). *Journal of the American Medical Association, 224,* 1415.

Cuthbertson, D., Smith, K., Babraj, J., et al. (2005). Anabolic signaling deficits underlie amino acid resistance of wasting, aging muscle. *FASEB Journal, 19,* 422–424.

Dangin, M., Guillet, C., Garcia-Rodena, C., et al. (2003). The rate of protein digestion affects protein gain differently during aging in humans. *Journal of Physiology, 549*(part 2), 635–644.

Davis, J. C., Bryan, S., Marra, C. A., et al. (2013). An economic evaluation of resistance training and aerobic training versus balance and toning exercises in older adults with mild cognitive impairment. *PLoS One, 8*(5), e63031. http://dx.doi.org/10.1371/journal.pone.0063031.

Davis, S. R., Castelo-Branco, C., Chedraui, P., et al. (2012). Understanding weight gain at menopause. *Climacteric, 15*(5), 419. http://dx.doi.org/10.3109/13697137.2012.707385.

Davis, W. J., Wood, D. T., Andrews, R. G., et al. (2008). Concurrent training enhances athletes' cardiovascular and cardiorespiratory measures. *Journal of Strength and Conditioning Research, 22*(5), 1503–1514.

Demling, R. H., & DeSanti, L. (2000). Effect of a hypocaloric diet, increased protein intake and resistance training on lean mass gains and fat mass loss in overweight police officers. *Annals of Nutrition and Metabolism, 44*(1), 21–29.

Déry, N., Pilgrim, M., Gibala, M., et al. (2013). Adult hippocampal neurogenesis reduces memory interference in humans: Opposing effects of aerobic exercise and depression. *Frontiers in Neuroscience, 7,* 66. http://dx.doi.org/10.3389/fnins.2013.00066.

Dhindsa, S. S., Batra, M., Kuhadiya, N. D., et al. (2013). Testosterone replacement decreases insulin resistance in hypogonadal men with type 2 diabetes. *Endocrine Reviews, 34*(03_MeetingAbstracts), OR22-1.

Dhurandhar, E. J., Dawson, J., Alcorn, A., Larsen, L. H., Thomas, E., Cardel, M., Bourland, A. C., Astrup, A., St-Onge, M., Hill, J. O., Apovian, C. M., Shikany, J., Allison, D. B. (2014). The effectiveness of breakfast recommendations on weight loss: A randomized controlled trial. *American Journal of Clinical Nutrition* (accepted for publication).

Duraffourd, et al. (2012, July 5). Mu-opioid receptors and dietary protein stimulate a gut-brain neural circuitry limiting food intake. *Cell.* http://dx.doi.org/10.1016/j.cell.2012.05.039.

Early, J. L., Apovian, C. M., Fernstrom, M. H., Greenway, F. A., Heber, D., Kushner, R. F., Cwik, K. M., Walch, J. K., Hewkin, A. C., & Blakesley, V. (2007). Sibutramine plus meal replacement therapy for body weight loss and maintenance in obese patients. *Obesity, 15,* 1464–1472.

Farb, M. G., Tiwari, S., Karki, S., Ngo, D. T., Carmine, B., Hess, D. T., Zuriaga, M. A., Walsh, K., Fetterman, J. L., Hamburg, N. M., Vita, J. A., Apovian, C. M., & Gokce, N. (2014, February). Cyclooxygenase inhibition improves endothelial vasomotor dysfunction of visceral adipose arterioles in human obesity. *Obesity (Silver Spring), 22*(2), 349–355. PMCID: PMC3766380.

Gagne, D. A., Vone Holle, A., Brownley, K. A., et al. (2012). Eating disorder symptoms and weight and shape concerns in a large web-based convenience sample of women ages 50 and above: Results of the gender and body image (GABI) study. *International Journal of Eating Disorders, 45*(7), 832–844. http://dx.doi.org/10.1002/eat.22030.

Gill, K. (2013, March 1). Centenarian's secret: Naples man turns 105, works out daily. NaplesNews.com.

Going, S. B. (2009). Osteoporosis and strength training. *American Journal of Lifestyle Medicine, 3*(4), 310–319. http://dx.doi.org/10.1177/1559827609334979. Retrieved from http://ajl.sagepub.com/content/3/4/310.short.

Heid, I. M., Jackson, A. U., Randall, J. C., et al. (2010). Meta-analysis identifies 13 new loci associated with waist-hip ratio and reveals sexual dimorphism in the genetic basis of fat distribution. *Nature Genetics, 42,* 949–960. Findings from the Genetic Investigation of Anthropometric Traits (GIANT).

Herber-Gast, G. C., & Mishra, G. D. (2013). Fruit, Mediterranean-style, and high-fat and -sugar diets are associated with the risk of night sweats and hot flushes in midlife: Results from a prospective cohort study. *American Journal of Clinical Nutrition, 97*(5), 1092–1099. http://dx.doi.org/10.3945/ajcn.112.049965.

Igel, L. I., Powell, A. G., Apovian, C. M., et al. (2012). Advances in medical therapy for weight loss and the weight-centric management of type 2 diabetes mellitus. *Current Atherosclerosis Reports, 14*(1), 60–69.

Imayama, I., Ulrich, C. M., Alfano, C. M., et al. (2012). Effects of a calorie restriction weight loss diet and exercise on inflammatory biomarkers in overweight/obese postmenopausal women: A randomized controlled trial. *Cancer Research, 72,* 2314–2326. http://dx.doi.org/10.1158/0008-5472.

Intermountain Medical Center. (2011, April 3). Routine periodic fasting is good for your health, and your heart, study suggests. *ScienceDaily.*

Islam, A., Civitarese, A. E., Hesslink, R. L., et al. (2012). Viscous dietary fiber reduces adiposity and plasma leptin and increases muscle expression of fat oxidation genes in rats. *Obesity, 20*(2), 349–355. http://dx.doi.org/10.1038/oby.2011.341.

Jensen, M. D., Ryan, D. H., Apovian, C. M., Ard, J. D., Comuzzie, A. G., Donato, K. A., Hu, F. B., Hubbard, V. S., Jakicic, J. M., Kushner, R. F., Loria, C. M., Millen, B. E., Nonas, C. A., Pi-Sunyer, F. X., Stevens, J., Stevens, V. J., Wadden, T. A., Wolfe, B. M., & Yanovski, S. Z. (2013, November 12). AHA/ACC/TOS guideline for the management of overweight and obesity in adults: A report of the American College of Cardiology/American Heart Association Task Force on Practice Guidelines and The Obesity Society. Advance online publication.

Layne, J. E., & Nelson, M. E. (1999). The effects of progressive resistance training on bone density: A review. *Medicine and Science in Sports and Exercise, 31*(1), 25–30.

Lovejoy, J. C., Champagne, C. M., de Jonge, L., et al. (2008). Increased visceral fat and decreased energy expenditure during the menopausal transition. *International Journal of Obesity, 32,* 949–958. http://dx.doi.org/10.1038/ijo.2008.25.

Maggio, M., Basaria, S., Ceda, G. P., et al. (2005). The relationship between testosterone and molecular markers of inflammation. *Journal of Endocrinological Investigation, 28*(11 Suppl Proceedings), 116–119.

Mavros, Y., Kay, S., Anderberg, K. A., et al. (2013). Changes in insulin resistance and HbA1c are related to exercise-mediated changes in body composition in older adults with type 2 diabetes. *Diabetes Care*. http://dx.doi.org/10.2337/dc12-2196.

McLafferty, C. L. Jr., Wetzstein, C. J., & Hunter, G. R. (2004). Resistance training is associated with improved mood in healthy older adults. *Perceptual and Motor Skills, 96*(3 part 1), 947–957.

Mehta, P. H., & Josephs, R. A. (2010). Testosterone and cortisol jointly regulate dominance: Evidence for a dual-hormone hypothesis. *Hormones and Behavior, 58*(5), 898–906. http://dx.doi.org/10.1016/j.yhbeh.2010.08.020.

Mosti, M. P., Kaehler, N., Stunes, A. K., et al. (2013). Maximal strength training in postmenopausal women with osteoporosis or osteopenia. *Journal of Strength and Conditioning Research, 27*(10), 2879–2886.

Paddon-Jones, D., & Rasmussen, B. B. (2009). Dietary protein recommendations and the prevention of sarcopenia: Protein, amino acid metabolism and therapy. *Current Opinion in Clinical Nutrition and Metabolic Care, 12*(1), 86–90. http://dx.doi.org/10.1097/MCO.0b013e32831cef8b.

Pasiakos, S. M., Cao, J. J., Margolis, L. M., et al. (2013). Effects of high-protein diets on fat-free mass and muscle protein synthesis following weight loss: A randomized controlled trial. *FASEB Journal, 27*(9), 3837–3847. http://dx.doi.org/10.1096/fj.13-230227.

Pi-Sunyer, X., Jensen, M., Ryan, D., Apovian, C. M., Millen, B., & Nonas, C. (2014, May). We stand by our guidelines. *Nature Reviews Endocrinology, 10*(5), 310.

Powell, A. G., Apovian, C. M., & Aronne, L. J. (2012). The combination of phentermine and topiramate is an effective adjunct to diet and lifestyle modification for weight loss and measures of comorbidity in overweight or obese adults with additional metabolic risk factors. *Evidence-Based Medicine, 17*(1), 14–15.

Pratley, R., Nicklas, B., Rubin, M., et al. (1994). Strength training increases resting metabolic rate and norepinephrine levels in healthy 50- to 65-year-old men. *Journal of Applied Physiology, 76*(1), 133–137.

Rantanen, T., Masaki, K., He, Q., et al. (2012). Midlife muscle strength and human longevity up to age 100 years: A 44-year prospective study among a decedent cohort. *Age (Dordr), 34*(3), 563–570. http://dx.doi.org/10.1007/s11357-011-9256-y.

Robinson, M. J., Burd, N.A., Breen, L., et al. (2013). Dose-dependent responses of myofibrillar protein synthesis with beef ingestion are enhanced with resistance exercise in middle-aged men. *Applied Physiology, Nutrition, and Metabolism, 38*(2), 120–125. http://dx.doi.org/10.1139/apnm-2012-0092.

Ruiz, J. R., Sui, X., Lobelo, F., et al. (2009). Muscular strength and adiposity as predictors of adulthood cancer mortality in men. *Cancer Epidemiology, Biomarkers & Prevention, 18*(5), 1468–1476.

Salam, R., Kshetrimayum, A. S., & Keisam, R. (2012). Testosterone and metabolic syndrome: The link. *Indian Journal of Endocrinology and Metabolism, 16* (Suppl 1), S12–S19. http://dx.doi.org/10.4103/2230-8210.94248.

Sieri, S., Krogh, V., Berrino, F., et al. (2010). Dietary glycemic load and index and risk of coronary heart disease in a large Italian cohort: The EPICOR study. *Archives of Internal Medicine, 170*(7), 640–647.

Srikanthan, P., & Karlamangla, A. S. (2011). Relative muscle mass is inversely associated with insulin resistance and prediabetes. Findings from The Third National Health and Nutrition Examination Survey. *Journal of Clinical Endocrinology & Metabolism, 96*(9), 2898–2903. http://dx.doi.org/10.1210/jc.2011-0435.

St-Onge, M. P., & Gallagher, D. (2010). Body composition changes with aging: The cause or the result of alterations in metabolic rate and macronutrient oxidation? *Nutrition, 26*(2), 152–155. http://dx.doi.org/10.1016/j.nut.2009.07.004.

University of Colorado–Boulder (2002, April 8). Vitamin C may help "juice up" metabolism in older adults, offsetting weight gain. *ScienceDaily.* Retrieved September 13, 2013.

Vincent, H. K., Bourguignon, C., & Vincent, K. R. (2006). Resistance training lowers exercise-induced oxidative stress and homocysteine levels in overweight and obese older adults. *Obesity, 14*(11), 1921–1930. http://dx.doi.org/10.1038/oby.2006.224.

Wang, L., Lee, I. M., Manson, J. E., et al. (2010). Alcohol consumption, weight gain, and risk of becoming overweight in middle-aged and older women. *Archives of Internal Medicine, 170*(5), 453–461. http://dx.doi.org/10.1001/archinternmed.2009.527.

West, D. N., Burd, N. A., Coffey, V. G., et al. (2011). Rapid aminoacidemia enhances myofibrillar protein synthesis and anabolic intramuscular signaling responses after resistance exercise. *American Journal of Clinical Nutrition, 94*(3), 795–803. http://dx.doi.org/10.3945/acjn.111.013722.

Westcott, W. (2009). ACSM strength training guidelines: Role in body composition and health enhancement. *ACSM's Health and Fitness Journal, 13*(4), 14–22. http://dx.doi.org/10.1249/FIT.0b013e3181aaf460.

Westcott, W. (2012). Resistance training is medicine: Effects of strength training on health. *Current Sports Medicine Reports, 11*(4), 209–216.

Wilson, M. E., Harshfield, G. A., Ortiz, L., et al. (2004). Relationship of body composition to stress-induced pressure natriuresis in youth. *American Journal of Hypertension, 17*(11 part 1), 1023–1028.

Index

About the Author

Just like many other college students, Caroline Apovian, MD, gained the freshman 10, which rapidly became the sophomore 15 and the junior 20. She studied nutrition and weight management in medical school, which helped turn her weight around and fueled the fire for her passion on helping others learn how to lose weight forever. Now one of the world's premier experts in the battle with weight loss, she distinguished herself as a leading researcher, treatment provider, and teacher in the field of weight loss while also working as director of the Nutrition and Weight Management Center at the Boston University Medical Center, director of Clinical Research at the Obesity Research Center of Boston University Medical Center, and professor of medicine at Boston University School of Medicine.

Her federal government positions include nutrition consultant to NASA and appointed member of the federal government's panel on the evaluation and treatment of overweight adults.

Her unparalleled accomplishments and tireless efforts in helping her patients have earned her recognition from her peers including the Physician Nutrition Specialist Award presented by the American Society of Clinical Nutrition for advancing nutrition education among doctors and medical students.

She is the recipient of major grants, including those from the NIH, the Atkins Foundation, and the Global Health Primary Care Initiative.

Dr. Apovian is a popular weight loss expert for EverydayHealth. com and is a medical adviser and a regular guest on *The Dr. Oz Show*.

A frequent national and international lecturer, Dr. Apovian has published papers, reviews, and book chapters on nutrition, obesity, and nutrition support and serves as manuscript reviewer for several prestigious journals, including *New England Journal of Medicine, Journal of Women's Health, International Journal of Obesity, Obesity Research, Digestive and Liver Disease,* and *Journal of Parenteral and Enteral Nutrition.*

Dr. Caroline Apovian lives in Waban, Massachusetts, with her husband and two sons. Her website is DrApovian.com and her Facebook page is www.facebook/drapovian.